THE 10 PRINCIPLES OF PERSONAL LONGEVITY

THE 10 PRINCIPLES OF PERSONAL LONGEVITY

MARTIN K. ETTINGTON

Copyright © 2022 by Martin K. Ettington

All rights reserved. No part of this publication may be reproduced, distributed, or transmitted in any form or by any means, including photocopying, recording, or other electronic or mechanical methods, without the prior written permission of the copyright owner and the publisher, except in the case of brief quotations embodied in critical reviews and certain other noncommercial uses permitted by copyright law. For permission requests, write to the publisher, addressed "Attention: Permissions Coordinator," at the address below.

ARPress
45 Dan Road Suite 5
Canton MA 02021

Hotline: 1(888) 821-0229
Fax: 1(508) 545-7580

Ordering Information:
Quantity sales. Special discounts are available on quantity purchases by corporations, associations, and others. For details, contact the publisher at the address above.

Printed in the United States of America.

ISBN-13:   Paperback   979-8-89389-821-7
              eBook   979-8-89389-822-4

Library of Congress Control Number: 2024923393

Table of Contents

1.0 Introduction 1

2.0 The Reality of Long Lived Persons 5

3.0 Defining Your Purpose in Life 33

4.0 Enabling Your Life Urge 43

5.0 The Importance of a Spiritual Connection 53

6.0 Having Love In Your Heart 65

7.0 Activate Your Vital Forces 95

8.0 The Science of Longevity 113

9.0 Keep your Physical Body Healthy 123

    Section A: Longevity Herbs and Supplements 123

    Section B: Long Lived Diets and Lifestyles 129

    Section C: Weight and Exercise 134

10.0 Using Your Intuition for Safety 137

11.0 Implementing the Ten Principles In Your Life 141

12.0 Summary 143

13.0 Bibliography 147

14.0 Index 151

The 10 Principles of Longevity are a holistic philosophy of long term health, greater happiness, and extended longevity which will change your life.

Written by well known internationally selling Author on Longevity Martin K. Ettington

These principles include the following:

- The Reality of Long Lived People
- Defining Your Purpose in Life
- Enabling the Life Urge
- Your Spiritual Health
- Having Love in Your Heart
- Energy Body Health
- The Science of Longevity
- Physical Body Health
- Using your Intuition for Safety
- Implementation of these principles

By following the principles in the book you will change your life forever and have a good chance of living to 150 years or older.

The 10 Principles of Personal Longevity

1) **Real Long Lived Persons Exist**
People really have lived a long time-so you can do it too

2) **Define Your Purpose in Life**
Know your life purpose-To live life with meaning

3) **Enable Your Life Urge**
Know without doubt that you will live a long and happy life

4) **The Importance of a Spiritual Connection**
A spiritual connection is important for happiness & long term health

5) **Having Love in your Heart**
Unconditional Love is is real-It will make you happier and healthier

6) **Activate your Vital Forces**
Improve the vitality of your energy body for health and to enjoy life more

7) **The Science of Longevity**
Use new therapies and discoveries from Science & Medicine

8) **Keep your Physical Body Healthy**
Eat a proper diet, use herbal supplements, and exercise

9) **Use Your Intuition for Safety**
Learn to use your intuition to keep you safe

10) **Implement the above principles in your life**
Implement these principles for long term health, greater happiness, and extended longevity

Formal Disclaimer

The author of this book is not a medical doctor, and the ideas contained herein may conflict with orthodox, mainstream medical opinion. The exercises, dietary measures, and other advice regarding health matters outlined in this book are not suitable for everyone, and under certain circumstances they could lead to injury.

You should not attempt self-diagnosis, and you should not embark on any exercise program, dietary regimen, or self-treatment of any kind without qualified medical supervision.

Nothing in this book should be construed as a promise of benefits or of results to be achieved, or a guarantee by the author or publisher of the safety or efficacy of its contents.

The author, the publisher, its editors, and its employees disclaim any liability, loss, or risk incurred directly or indirectly as a result of the use or application of any of the contents of this book.

Other books by Martin K. Ettington

Spiritual and Metaphysics Books:

Prophecy: A History and How to Guide God Like Powers and Abilities Enlightenment for Newbies
Removing Illusions to Find True Happiness
Using the Scientific Method to Study the Paranormal
A Compendium of Metaphysics and How to Guides (Six books together in one volume)
Love from the Heart
The Enlightenment Experience Learn Your Soul's Purpose Pursuing Enlightenment
A Modern Man's Search for Truth
Use Intuition and Prophecy to Improve Your Life The Handbook of Spiritual and Energy Healing Pure Spirituality and God

Longevity & Immortality:

Physical Immortality: A History and How to Guide The Commentaries of Living Immortals
Records of Extremely Long Lived Persons Enlightenment and Immortality
Longevity Improvements from Science The 10 Principles of Personal Longevity Telomeres & Longevity
The Diets and Lifestyles of the World's Oldest Peoples The Longevity Six Books Bundle
Long Lived Plants and Animals

Science Fiction:

Out of This Universe
The Immortals of the Interstellar Colony The Mystic Soldier
The Immortality Sci Fi Bundle Visiting Many Universes
The History of Science Fiction and Fantasy

The God Like Powers Series:

Human Invisibility Invulnerability and Shielding Teleportation
Psychokinesis
Our Energy Body, Auras, and Thoughtforms The God Like Powers Series—Volume 1 Compilation

The Yoga Discovery Series:

Yoga-An Ancient Art Form
Hatha Yoga-Helping you Live Better Raja Yoga-Through the Ages
The Yoga Discovery Package

Business & Coaching Books:

Creating, Publishing, & Marketing Practitioner eBooks Building a Successful Longevity Coaching Business Why Become a Coach?
The Professional Coaching Success Trilogy 2020-Make Money Writing and Selling Books
The 2020 Handbook of High Paying Work Without a College Degree The important of Creativity and How to Improve Yours

Science, Technology, and Misc.

Future Predictions By and Engineer & Seer The Unusual Science & Technology Bundle The Real Atlantis-In the Eye of the Sahara
Removing Limits On Our Consciousness-And Thinking Outside the Box
Universal Holistic Philosophy

Survival

Survival of Humanity Throughout the Ages 33 Incredible True Survival Stories
The Importance of Fire in History and Mythology
How to Survive Anything: From the Wilderness to Man Made Disasters
Building and Stocking a Nuclear Shelter for less than $10,000 The Human Survival Five Books Bundle

Legendary Beings

Are Cryptozoological Animals Real or Imaginary? Fire in History and Mythology
All About Dragons
Sea Serpents and Ocean Monsters
The Legendary Animals Five Books Bundle The Mythical People of Ireland

Ancient History

The Real Atlantis-In the Eye of the Sahara Ancient & Prehistoric Civilizations
Ancient & Prehistoric Civilizations-Book Two The History of Antediluvian Giants
The Antediluvian History of Earth Ancient Underground Cities and Tunnels Strange Objects Which Should Not Exist More Out of Place Artifacts
Strange and Ancient Places in the USA
A Theory of Ancient Prehistory And Giant Aliens The Destruction of Civilization About 10,500 B.C. A Timeline of Intelligent Life on Earth

Aliens and Space

Aliens and Secret Technology Aliens Are Already Among Us
Designing and Building Space Colonies Humanity and the Universe
All About Moon Bases
All About Mars Journeys and Settlement The Space and Aliens Six Books Bundle
A Theory of Ancient Prehistory and Giant Aliens
The Space Colonies and Space Structures Coloring Book All About Asteroids
Spaceships, Past, Present, and Future
Astronauts, Cosmonauts, and Other Important Space Flyers All About Mars Journeys and Settlement
Mining the Asteroid Belt

Time Travel and Dimensions

Real Time Travel Stories From a Psychic Engineer
The Real Nature of Time: An Analysis of Physics, Prophecy, and Time Travel Experiences
Stories of Parallel Dimensions
We Live in a Malleable Reality-and We Can Change It

The Longevity Training Series

(A transcription of the online Multimedia Longevity Coaching Training Program)

The Personal Longevity Training Series-Book1-Long Lived Persons
The Personal Longevity Training Series-Book2-Your Soul's Purpose
The Personal Longevity Training Series-Book3-Enable Your Life Urge
The Personal Longevity Training Series-Book4-Your Spiritual Connection
The Personal Longevity Training Series-Book5-Having Love in Your Heart
The Personal Longevity Training Series-Book6-Energy Body Health
The Personal Longevity Training Series-Book7-The Science of Longevity
The Personal Longevity Training Series-Book8-Physical Body Health
The Personal Longevity Training Series-Book9-Avoiding Accidents
The Personal Longevity Training Series-Book10-Implementing These Principles

The Personal Longevity Training Series-Books One Thru Ten

These books are all available in digital and printed formats from my website and on Amazon, Barnes & Noble, Apple iTunes, and many other sites

My Books Website is: http://mkettingtonbooks.com

Signup for our Mailing List to get the following:

1. A discount coupon for 25% discount on all books on our site
2. Occasional Notices of new books available
3. Occasional Email on other offerings of ours (Monthly) Go to this link to sign-up:

http://personal-longevity.com/mkebooks/emailsignup/

And click this link to get the FREE 102 page eBook titled

"Secrets of Many Things"

If you have any questions about this book or other subjects please contact the Author at:

mke@mkettingtonbooks.com

Book Dedication

This book is dedicated to everyone who feels that they want more time to live their life and enjoy it to the fullest.

We limit ourselves as to what is possible in our lives.

My hope is that this book will help you breakout of your "reality box" and live to your full potential longevity and accomplishment in life.

1.0 Introduction

They say that one's mission in life can often be shown to be pre-ordained by an event that happens when you are very young.

This may have happened to me when I was about four years old.

I lived in upstate New York and my Mom used to sometimes take me to Harris Hill near Elmira to ride the ponies.

Harris Hill was also the glider capital of the world and sometimes we would stop at the field to watch the gliders taking off.

One day I was standing on the concrete near the hangers and saw a grey haired tall man talking to some women.

I had a strange feeling and I don't know why I did this, but I wandered over to him and said "Are you the man who never dies?".

He gave me a very strange look and then my mother grabbed me and took me away apologizing for me.

Many years later I read that a man who may be as much as a thousand years old lived in that area. So who knows who I met that day.

****

In September of 2008 I wanted to write a book to give back much of what I had learned over the years about spiritual development and metaphysics.

In looking for a topic I was fascinated by the claims of many Indian Yogis that were said to live hundreds of years. I wondered if these claims were true and this was really possible.

This led to my research on long lived people and what I found was shocking. I found pictures, bios, and videos of people all over the world that had lived and were living well beyond the age of 150 years. I even found one Chinese man who was claimed to have lived to 256 years old. (Li Ching Yun who you will learn more about later)

As an engineer and career IT consultant I also have an analytical side and wanted to understand and explain extreme longevity to others.

The result of my research and meditations was my first book on longevity titled "Physical Immortality: A History and How to Guide".

That book led to my networking with a lot of persons in the extreme longevity movement. Many of them are called "Immortalists" since they follow practices they believe will lead to their own life extension.

I also researched and wrote more books on related spiritual and holistic health topics over the last five years as I continued to learn and grow.

In mid 2012, I took all of the knowledge I had been accumulating and started to develop a new approach to teaching people about the possibilities of long term health, greater happiness, and extended longevity.

This led me to codifying my ten principles of personal longevity which are the following:

- The Reality of Long Lived People
- Defining Your Purpose in Life
- Enabling the Life Urge
- Your Spiritual Health
- Having Love in Your Heart
- Energy Body Health
- The Science of Longevity
- Physical Body Health
- Using your Intuition for Safety
- Implementation of these principles

Each principle is a progressive step towards helping the individual to maximize their long term health which leads towards extended longevity.

The rest of this book is designed to elaborate these ten principles with evidence, theory, and exercises to help everyone live as healthy, happy, and as long a life as possible.

I am also developing my business in parallel with this book to help everyone implement these principles in their lives.

As of 2017 we offer these services to everyone regarding longevity:

- Longevity Coaching and Certification Programs-To provide new skills to professional wellness coaches and additional skills to other wellness professionals.
- Packaged Longevity Workshops--For business to integrate their wellness programs together and teach clients about the 10 Principles in detail

You can learn more details about all that we do at our website:

> http://personal-longevity.com

2.0 The Reality of Long Lived Persons

The first principle of personal longevity is to understand that there are many records of very long lived people.

People on this planet having been living to very great ages back before records were ever kept and you need to know this information to understand that you can do it too.

Considering the skepticism with which most people view records of very long lifetimes, I thought it would be useful to compile a list of as many long lived persons as possible; to show that these records exist and people really have lived lives of extraordinary length.

Nothing will convince somebody who has a closed mind or has to see the person's making these claims themselves. However, this list may start most people questioning that what they have been told all their lives about the limits to living; which are completely wrong.

Most of the persons listed were either from Europe, or North and South America.

I think the reason for this is that records have been better kept in the West in recent centuries. There were most probably as many persons living in Africa and Asia who lived long lives—we just don't have their records.

Also included in this chapter is a section on unbelievably long lived people to show that the possible length of physical life may be much longer than any of us can imagine; I.E. 9,000 years.

Below is a list from several sources which can be verified by going to the original records.

Records of numerous long lived individuals:

Ages 110-119

From the Immortality Article:

Of interest to Americans is the case of David Kinnison, who, when one hundred and eleven, related to Lossing the historian the tale of the Boston Tea Party, of which he had been a member.

Anthony Senish, a farmer of the village of Limoges, died in 1770 in his one hundred and eleventh year. He labored until two weeks before his death, had still his hair, and his sight had not failed him. His usual food was chestnuts and Turkish corn; he had never been bled or used any medicine.

Not very long ago there was alive in Tacony, near Philadelphia, a shoemaker named R. Glen in his one hundred and fourteenth year. He had seen King William III, and all his faculties were perfectly retained; he enjoyed good health, walking weekly to Philadelphia to church. His third wife was but thirty years old.

He died in good mental condition at the age of one hundred and fifteen.

The census of 1864 for the town of Pilaguin, Ecuador, lying 11,000 feet above the level of the sea and consisting of about 2000 inhabitants, gives 100 above seventy, 30 above ninety, five above one hundred, and one at <u>one hundred and fifteen years.</u>

Longevity in Ireland. Lord Bacon said that at one time there was not a village in all Ireland in which there was not a man living upward of eighty. In Dunsford, a small village, there were living at one time 80 persons above the age of four score.

Ages 120-129

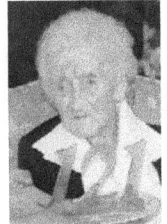
The oldest age that the Guinness Book of World Records recognizes is Jeanne Louise Calment (21 February 1875 – 4 August 1997, 10:45 CET). She had the longest confirmed human life span in history, living 122 years and 164 days (44,724 days total). She lived in Arles, France, for her entire life, and outlived both her daughter and grandson. (And who appointed Guinness as the final word on longevity?—Nobody did)

From the Immortality Article:

Eglebert Hoff was a lad driving a team in Norway when the news was brought that Charles I was beheaded. He died in Fishkill, N.Y., in 1764 at the age of one hundred and twenty-eight. He never used spectacles, read fluently, and his memory and senses were retained until his death, which was due to an accident.

Ages 130-139

From the Immortality Article:

There was a man by the name of Butler who died at Kilkenny in 1769 aged one hundred and thirty- three.

Time, 14 July, 1967; Toronto Star, 19 Sept. & 2 Oct., 1972; 13 May, 1976:

Charlie Smith was 133 in 1976 in the state of Florida, USA. Born in Africa and brought to States as a slave at 12, he worked steadily picking fruit until 113. In 1976 he received an honorary diploma from Polk County School System, though he had little formal schooling.

South Africa-Moloko Temo (4 July 1874? - 2 or 3 June 2009) died in South Africa at the alleged age of 134, which would put her birth in the Transvaal.

Nicolas Petours, curate of the parish of Baleene and afterward canon of the Cathedral of Constance, died at the age of one hundred and thirty-seven; he was always a healthy, vigorous man, and celebrated mass five days before his death.

In the State of Vera Cruz, Mexico, as late as 1893 a man died at the age of one hundred and thirty- seven.

Mr. Evans of Spital Street, Spitalfields, London, died in 1780 aged one hundred and thirty-nine, having full possession of his mental faculties.

Ages 140-149

Among the Mission Indians of Southern California there are reported instances of longevity ranging from one hundred and twenty to one hundred and forty.

Lieutenant Gibbons found in a village in Peru one hundred inhabitants who were past the century mark, and another credible explorer in the same territory records a case of longevity of one hundred and forty. This man was very temperate and always ate his food cold, partaking of meat only in the middle of the day.

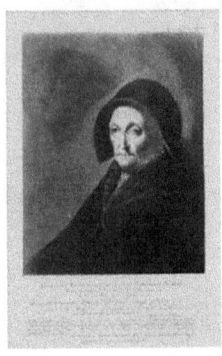
Katherine Fitzgerald (1464?-1604), 140, Ireland's Nathaniel Grogan's 1806 engraving of Lord Kerry's portrait of Katherine FitzGerald, Countess of Desmond is on the left.

Lady Desmond was reported to have been capable, just before her death, of walking every week to her local market town, a distance of 4–5 miles, and it was said that all her teeth had been renewed a few years earlier. Her death was caused when she fell from a tree while picking cherries.

Dr. William Hotchkiss, said to have reached the age of one hundred and forty years, died in St. Louis April 1, 1895. He went to St. Louis forty years ago, and has always been known as the "color doctor." In his peculiar practice of medicine he termed his patients members of his "circles," and claimed to treat them by a magnetic process. Dr. A. J. Buck says that his Masonic record has been traced back one hundred years, showing conclusively that he was one hundred and twenty-one years old. A letter received from his old home in Virginia, over a year ago, says that he was born there in 1755.

Mrs. Eckelston, a widow in Phillipstown, Kings County, Ireland, died in 1690 at one hundred and forty- three.

Jean Effingham died in Cornwall in 1757 in his one hundred and forty-fourth year. He was born in the reign of James I, and was a soldier at the battle of Hochstadt. He never drank strong liquors and rarely ate meat. Eight days before his death he walked three miles.

Colonel Thomas Winslow was supposed to have died in Ireland on August 26, 1766, aged one hundred and forty-six. He rode after the hounds while yet a centenarian.

Ages 150-159

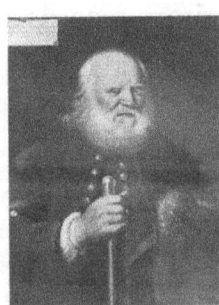
Christian Jacobsen Drakenberg died at 150 years in 1772. A sailor for 91 years, he fought in the war against the Swedes, then became a merchant seaman. In 1694, he was taken prisoner by Algerian pirates but set free after 15 years of slavery, he resumed his life as a seaman. In 1737, at the age of 110, he married a widow of 60 years. He was known as 'the old man of the north'.

Even in old age Drakenberg was bursting with strength. Whoever would shake his hand, never forgot the experience and ventured no second attempt. It was reported that after death his body mummified and did not rot. (Similar to reports on Yogananda)

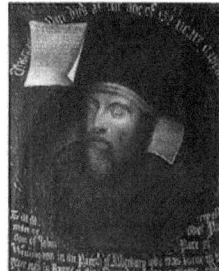

In the chancel of the Honigton Church, Wiltshire, is a black marble monument to the memory of G. Stanley, a gentleman, who died in 1719, aged one hundred and fifty- one.

And in Acsadi & Nemeskeri, p.17 & Toronto Evening Telegram, 9 Sept., 1939; 26 April, 1942. (Also in the Longevity Article)

Thomas Parr, 152, died 1635, in England. Thomas Parr (or Parre), among Englishmen known as "old Parr," was a poor farmer's servant, born in 1483. He remained single until eighty. His first wife lived thirty-two years, and eight years after her death, at the age of one hundred and twenty, he married again. Until his one hundred and thirtieth year he performed his ordinary duties, and at this age was even accustomed to thresh.

He was visited by Thomas, Earl of Arundel and Surrey, and was persuaded to visit the King in London. His intelligence and venerable demeanor impressed everyone, and crowds thronged to see him and pay homage. The journey to London, together with the excitement and change in mode of living, undoubtedly hastened his death, which occurred in less than a year. He was one hundred and fifty-two years and nine months old, and had lived under nine Kings of England. Harvey examined his body and at the necropsy his internal organs were found in a most perfect state. His cartilages were not even ossified, as is the case generally with the very aged. The slightest cause of death could not be discovered, and the general impression was that he died from being over-fed and too-well treated in London. His great-grandson was said to have died in this century in Cork at the age of one hundred and three. Parr is celebrated by a monument reared to his memory in Westminster Abbey.

San Francisco Chronicle, 21 Jan., 1969, p.15:

Sampson Skakoragaro is 158 in and living in Tanzania, Africa. In 1969 he had a successful cataract operation and "was in high spirits and talkative". He had fathered his youngest son at 136. Married in 1934 at age 123, with sons born in 1935, 1941, and 1945, the two eldest are teachers and the youngest a tailor. He has had three wives and 16 children. He himself was the eldest of 58 sons. His father lived to 123 years, had 39 wives, and 45 daughters.

Ages 160-169

From the Sear's Wonders of the World we have this one:

"December 5, 1830, died at St. Andrews, Jamaica, the property of Sir Edward Hyde East, Robert Lynch, a black slave in comfortable circumstances, who perfectly recollected the great earthquake of 1692, and further recollected the person and equipages of the lieutenant-governor, Sir Henry Morgan, whose third and last governorship commenced in 1680, viz., one hundred and fifty years before.

Allowing for this early recollection the age of ten years, this black must have died at the age of one hundred and sixty years."

Huteland speaks of Joseph Surrington, who died near Bergen, Norway, at the age of one hundred and sixty. Marvelous to relate, he had one living son of one hundred and three and another of nine. There was a Polish peasant who reached one hundred and fifty-seven and had constantly labored up to his one hundred and forty-fifth year, always clad lightly, even in cold weather. Voigt admits the extreme age of one hundred and sixty.

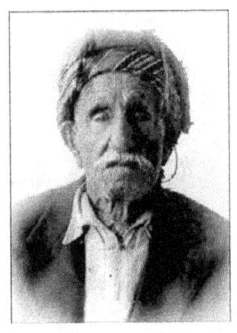
Zaro Ağa Mutki, Bitlis, Ottoman Empire, Born in 1774 or 1777 İstanbul, Turkey, 29 June 1934, a Kurdish man named Zaro Ağa died in the United States in 1933 at the age of 164 years. According to the death certificate given by his Doctor, Zaro Ağa's age was 157. He died in Istanbul, although there exists some confusion about the death place, Probably because the body was sent to the U.S. right after his death. He was born in Bitlis, and lived Mutki, Gundê Meydan, Kurdish, Ottoman Turkey, worked as a construction worker when he was young; then moved to Istanbul where he worked as a porter for more than 100 years and finally retired as a janitor.

He was a major attraction to press during his last years as the world's oldest living man and one who had traveled to many countries, including the United States, the United Kingdom, Italy and France.

"Jonas Warren of Balydole died in 1787 aged one hundred and sixty-seven. He was called the "father of the fisherman" in his vicinity, as he followed the trade for ninety-five years."

There was a woman living in Moscow in 1848 who was said to be <u>one hundred and sixty-eight</u>; she had been married five times and was one hundred and twenty-one at her last wedding. D'Azara records the age of one hundred and eighty, and Roequefort speaks of two cases at one hundred and fifty.

From the "Anomalies and Curiosities of Medicine Part 1" are found these interesting references:

In a churchyard near Cardiff, Glamorganshire, is the following inscription: "Here lieth the body of William Edwards, of Caereg, who departed this life 24th February, Anno Domini 1668, anno aetatis suae one hundred and sixty-eight"

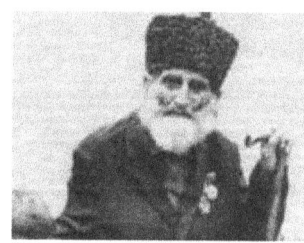

Of course who could forget Shirali Mislimov! There are many references to Shirali Mislimov including the January 1972 issue of National Geographic. However from Toronto Evening Telegram, 20 May, 1971 & the Ottawa Citizen, 13 Feb., 1967, p.18 & Life, 16 Sept.,1966, p.121 & Gris & Merlin, p.88-115 & Time, 17 Sept., 1973 we have this:

Shirali Mislimov, 168, Died 1973, in Azerbaijan, USSR.

On his birthday (1971) he rose at dawn to do his daily chores in the garden and orchard. Among his well-wishers were doctors who gave him his annual physical and judged his health perfect. He has never been ill, though forced to give up riding horseback recently.

At 160 he journeyed to the capital city (his first visit). There a doctor recorded his pulse at 72 and blood pressure at 120/75, and this was after a three story climb! He neither smoked or drank.

Survived by his third wife, 107 years old, 219 other family members, including a grandchild aged 100 years.

From the Longevity article we have:

Henry Jenkins, 169, died 1670, in Yorkshire England.

Possibly the most celebrated case of longevity on record is that of Henry Jenkins. This remarkable old man was born in Yorkshire in 1501 and died in 1670, aged one hundred and sixty-nine. He remembered the battle of Flodden Field in 1513, at which time he was twelve years old.

It was proved from the registers of the Chancery and other courts that he had appeared in evidence one hundred and forty years before his death and had had an oath administered to him. In the office of the King's Remembrancer is a record of a deposition in which he appears as a witness at one hundred and fifty-seven. When above one hundred he was able to swim a rapid stream.

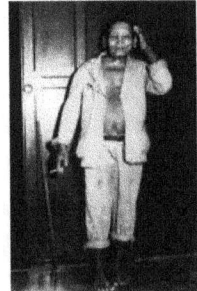 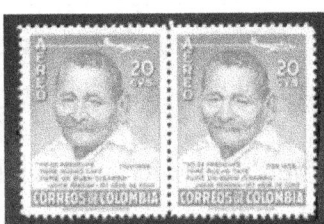 From Toronto Star Weekly Mag.,15 Dec.,1956, p.2f & Time, 14 April, 1958, p.88.:

Javier Pereira, 169, died 1958, in Columbia, S.A. Only 4'4" tall, weighed 75 pounds. Taken to New York Hospital Cornell Medical Centre in 1956. At that time he had all his hair without any gray, teeth were all gone, skin

like old brown wrinkled leather, eyes cloudy but still serviceable, hands arthritic but a powerful hand-shake firm and surprisingly youthful. Arteries showed no signs at all of

deterioration. His endurance and feats were remarkable like standing on one leg and pirouetting without losing his balance, walking three blocks and climbing two flights of stairs without losing his breath. He had no immediate relatives (though married 5 times), his last grandchild had died 15 years ago at age 85 years. He was known by oldsters in his own village when they were in their teens as

the "old Indian who liked to dance". <u>Ages 170-179</u>

From Prichard, p.12 & Acsadi & Nemeskeri, p.16. we have this one:

John Rovin, 172, died 1741, in Temesvar, Hungry. His wife, Sarah Desson Rovin died the same year at the age of 164 after a marriage of 147 years.

2.0 The Reality of Long Lived Persons

From the Toronto Daily Star, 15 Dec. 1952 we have this one:

Baba Harainsingh, 176, died 1952, in India.

He had grown a complete set of teeth, the previous ones having fallen out when he was about 100 in the 1870s, his gray hair was also turning black again!

Elizabeth Yorath wife of Edmund Thomas was buried the 13th of February 1668, aged 177. <u>Ages 180-189</u>

"LLANMAES, or LLANVAES (LLAN-MAES), a parish in the hundred of COWBRIDGE, county of GLAMORGAN, SOUTH WALES, 3 1/2 miles (S.) from Cowbridge, containing 234 inhabitants. The salubrity of the air is attested by several entries in the parish register of the burial of persons whose lives had been extended to an almost incredibly protracted period. Among these, the most remarkable are the following, which have been extracted verbatim" Ivan Yorath buried a Saturday the XVII day of July anno doni 1621 et anno regni regis vicessimo primo annoque aetatis circa 180. He was a Sowdiar in the fights of Boswoorthe, and lived at Lantwit Major, and he lived much by fishing.

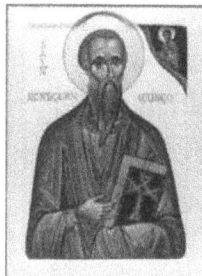

From Acsadi & Nemeskeri, p.16 we have more:

Kentigren, 185, died 5 Jan. 600 A.D. in Scotland. He was the founder of Glasgow Abbey. The legends that grew up around Saint Kentigern include stories of many miracles, some of which are illustrated on the Glasgow City coat of arms.

There is even the story of an encounter with King Arthur's wizard, Merlin, who is said to have become a Christian and been baptized by Kentigren.

This item is referenced in "Acsadi & Nemekeri", P. 16 & Baily, 1857 (And in the Longevity Article):

Petratsh Zartan (Setrasch Czartan) died 1724 in Hungry at the age of 187; Setrasch Czarten, or, as he is called by Baily, Petratsh Zartan, was born in Hungary at a village four miles from Teneswaer in 1537. He lived for one hundred and eighty years in one village; and died at the age of one hundred and eighty-seven, or, as another authority has it, one hundred and eighty-five.

A few days before his death he had walked a mile to wait at the post-office for the arrival of travelers and to ask for succor, which on account of his remarkable age, was rarely refused him. He had lost nearly all his teeth and his beard and hair were white. He was accustomed to eat a little cake the Hungarians call kalatschen, with which he drank milk. After each repast he took a glass of eau-de-vie. His son was living at ninety-seven and his descendants to the fifth generation embellished his old age.

Shortly before his death Count Wallis had his portrait painted. Comparing his age with that of others, we find that he was five years older than the Patriarch Isaac, ten more than Abraham, thirty-seven more than Nahor, sixteen more than Henry Jenkins, and thirty-three more than "old Parr."

Age 192

There has been recently reported from Vera Cruz, Mexico, in the town of Teluca, where the registers are carefully and efficiently kept, the death of a man one hundred and ninety-two years old.

Age 207

Another interesting item from "Museum Eurpeaum" published in 1825:

"The most remarkable instance of longevity which we meet with in British history is that of Thomas Carn, who, according to the parish register of St. Leonard, Shoreditch, died 28th January, 1588 at the astonishing age of two hundred and seven years!

He was born in the reign of Richard the Second, anno 1381, and lived in the reigns of twelve kings and queens, Richard II, Henry IV, V, and VI. Edward IV and V, Richard III, Henry VII and VIII, Edward, VI, Mary, and Elizabeth.

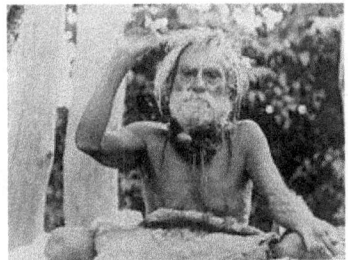

The veracity of the above may be readily observed by any person who chooses to consult the above mentioned register."

Age 250

Devraha Baba was a hermit from Vrindavan Claimed to have been 250 years old at his death in May 1990. He was considered to be a "spiritual guide to everyone from a pauper to the most powerful... above narrow confines of caste and community. "Village people as well as important personalities waited for hours to have a glimpse or *darshan* of him. He received visits from politicians seeking his blessings at the time of general elections, including Indira Gandhi, Buta Singh, and Rajiv Gandhi. Rajiv Gandhi and his wife Sonia Gandhi visited his ashram on the eve of the 1989 elections. He used to bless the devotees with his feet.

He lived on a 12-foot-high (3.7 m) wooden platform near the river and wore a small deerskin. A barricade of wooden planks hid his semi-naked body from his devotees, and he came down only to bathe in the river. (A video can be found of him on YouTube)

LI CHING-YUN: The Longest Lived person of record-256 Years

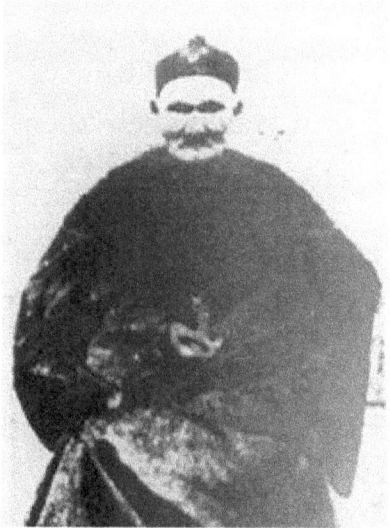

Below is an excerpt of an article from the New York Times (10): The New York Times, Saturday, May 6, 1933

LI CHING-YUN DEAD; GAVE HIS AGE AS 197

"Keep Quiet heart, Sit Like a Tortoise, Sleep Like a Dog," His advice for a Long Life. Inquiry Put Age At 256.

Reported to have buried 23 wives and had 180 descendents – sold herbs for first 100 years.

Peiping, May 5 – Li Ching-Yun, a resident of Kaihsien, in the Province of Szechwan, who contended that he was one of the world's oldest men and said he was born in 1736 – which would make him 197 years old – died today.

A Chinese dispatch from Chungking telling of Mr. Li's death said he attributed his longevity to peace of mind and that it was his belief everyone could live at least a century by attaining inward calm.

Compared with estimates of Li Ching-Yun's age in previous reports from China, the above dispatch is conservative. In 1930 it was said Professor Wu Chung-chien, dean of the department of Education in Minkuo University, had found records showing Li was born in 1677 and that Imperial Chinese Government congratulated him on his 150th and 200th birthdays.

A correspondent of The New York Times wrote in 1928 that many of the oldest men in Li's neighborhood asserted their grandfathers knew him as boys and that he was then a grown man.

According to the generally accepted tales told in his province. Li was able to read and write as a child, and by his tenth birthday had traveled in Kansu, Shansi, Tibet, Annam, Siam and Manchuria

gathering herbs. For the first hundred years he continued at this occupation. Then he switched to selling herbs gathered by others.

Wu Pei-fu, the warlord, took Li into his house to learn the secret of living to 250. Another pupil said Li told him to "keep a quiet heart, sit like a tortoise, walk sprightly like a pigeon and sleep like a dog."

According to one version of Li's married life he had buried away twenty-three wives and was living with his twenty-fourth, a woman of '60.' Another account, which in 1928 credited him with 180 living descendents, comprising eleven generations, recorded only fourteen marriages. This second authority said his eyesight was good; also, that the fingernails of his right hand were very long, and "long" for a Chinese might mean longer than any finger nails ever dreamed of in the United States.

One statement of The Times correspondent which probably caused skeptical readers to believe Li was born more recently that 1677, was that "many who have seen him recently declare that his facial appearance is no different from that of persons two centuries his junior."

An article from the May 15, 1933 issue of Time magazine titled:

Tortoise-Pigeon-Dog

In the province of Szechwan in China lived until last week Li Ching-Yun By his own story he was

born in 1736, had lived 197 years. By the time he was ten years old he had traveled in Kansu, Shansi, Tibet, Annam, Siam and Manchuria gathering herbs. Some said he had buried 23 wives, was living with his 24th. a woman of 60, had descendants of eleven generations. The fingernails of his venerable right hand were six inches long. Yet to skeptical Western eyes he looked much like any Chinese 60-year-old. In 1930 Professor Wu Chung-chieh, dean of the department of education at Chengtu University, found records that the Imperial Chinese Government had congratulated one Li Ching-yun in 1827 on his birthday. The birthday was his 150th, making the man who died last week— if it was the same Li Ching-yun, and respectful Chinese preferred to think so—a 256-year-old.

More about Li Chang Yun from the *Toronto Evening Telegram*, 26 April, 1942: LI CHING-YUN, *256, died May, 1933, Szechun Province, China.*

At the age of 100 he was awarded by the Chinese Government a special Honor Citation for extraordinary services to his country. This document is available in existing archives. It is reported that he gave a series of 28 lectures at the University of Sinkiang when he was over 200 years old. He attributed his longevity to his life-long vegetarian diet and regular use of rejuvenating herbs plus "inward calm".

A renowned herbalist, he used Fo-ti-tieng and ginseng daily in the form of tea. He enjoyed excellent health, outlived 23 wives, and kept his own natural teeth and hair. Those who saw him at age of 200 testified that he did not appear much older than a man in his fifties.

A researched Li Chang (Ching) Yun is featured in this 1980 book: "The Seed of the Woman" by Arthur C. Custance.

Li Ching Yun is also featured in the recent book: "Qigong Teachings of a Taoist Immortal: The Eight Essential Exercises of Master Li Ching-Yun" by Stuart Alve Olson.

Recent Reports of Living Extremely long lived persons

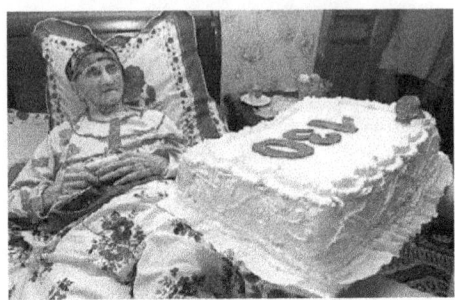

A recent report on a Long Lived Woman who is alive and 130 years old-

By MISHA DZHINDZHIKHASHVILI, Associated Press Writer 7/8/10:

SACHIRE, Georgia – Authorities in the former Soviet republic of Georgia claim a woman from a remote mountain village turned 130 on Thursday, making her the oldest person on Earth.

Antisa Khvichava from western Georgia was born on July 8, 1880, said Georgiy Meurnishvili, spokesman for the civil registry at the Justice Ministry.

The woman, who lives with her 40-year-old grandson in an idyllic vine-covered country house in the mountains, retired from her job as a tea and corn picker in 1965, when she was 85, records say.

"I've always been healthy, and I've worked all my life — at home and at the farm," said Khvichava, in a bright dress and headscarf, her withering lips rejuvenated by shiny red lipstick. Sitting in the chair and holding her cane, Khvichava spoke quietly through an interpreter since she never went to school to learn Georgian and speaks only the local language, Mingrelian.

But Meurnishvili showed two Soviet-era documents that he says attest to her age. Scores of officials, neighbors, friends, and descendants backed up her claim as the world's top senior.

A 157 Year old woman named Turinah in Sumatra:

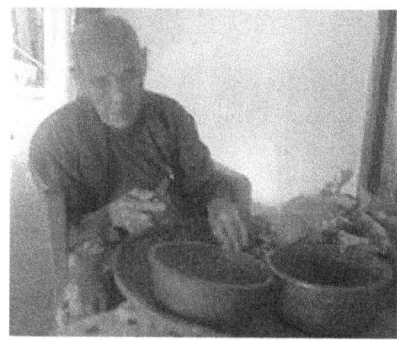

(ABC News Australia-Posted Mon Jun 7, 2010 10:23pm AEST):

Census officials have said they believe the woman's claims to have been born in 1853, when Giuseppe Verdi's La Traviata debuted in Venice, the Crimean War erupted and San Francisco got its first street signs at intersections. (Born June 7, 1853).

"There's no authentic data to prove her age, but judging from her statements and the age of her adopted daughter, who's now 108 years old, it's difficult to doubt it," statistics bureau official Jhonny Sardjono said Monday.

South Sumatran villager Turinah would be fully 35 years older than Calment (Jeanne Calment, who died in 1997 at the age of 122) according to officials. Mr. Sardjono said "Even more incredible, she still works around the house and has smoked clove cigarettes all her life".

"Despite her age she still has an incredible memory, clear sight and has no hearing problems. She speaks Dutch quite fluently," he said.

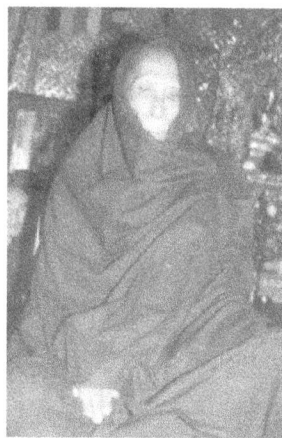

The Oldest Man Alive Today?

I published a short posting in 2013 on the book "Wonders of Mebegon Village" about some Buddhists in Burma who are living to extraordinary ages.

However, due to the rarity of the book I don't think readers really got the import of what I was saying.

The picture above is of Wizzardo (Siddha) Sayadaw U. Kowida who was born in the year 908 A.D. and who is still alive. He went through a fire transformation ceremony to achieve his immortality.

His community believes in an alchemical transformation process that allows them to live to extraordinary ages after also achieving certain levels of enlightenment.

We have heard rumors of other people living to hundreds of years old but this is the first picture I've ever seen of somebody who is purportedly this old.

This is a big deal! I have a very extensive library of evidence of long lived persons but no pictures of anyone else more than 300 years old.

Some of his followers also are hundreds of years old and they live in a small community in a remote part of Burma.

I know it sounds ridiculous, but after all of the evidence I've seen of long lived persons over the years this is just another point of data showing that we all have the potential for extreme longevity if we would only believe it's possible and take the appropriate actions.

This next couple of sections are undocumented stories of what may be possible longevity histories— but are pretty far out—we don't really know enough to say that these stories are true. But what if they are?

How about these long lived person claims?

Trailanga Swami (also Trailinga Swami, Ganapati Saraswati) (reportedly c. 1529 or 1607 -1887) was a Hindu yogi famed for his spiritual powers who lived in Varanasi, India. He is regarded as a legendary figure in Bengal, with many stories told about his yogic powers and longevity.

According to some accounts, Trailanga Swami lived to be around 300 years old, residing at Varanasi between 1737-1887. He is regarded as an incarnation of God Shiva, and Ramakrishna. A contemporary Bengali saint referred to him as the "The Walking Shiva of Varanasi".

According to the county annals of Yong Tai in Fujian Province, Chen Jun was born in the first year of Zhong He time (881 AD) under the reign of Emperor Xi Zong during the Tang Dynasty. He died in the Tai Ding time of the Yuan Dynasty (1324 AD), after living for 443 years. During the course of his lifetime he allegedly had 23 wives and about 200 descendants.

The ancient Greek author Lucian is the presumed author of *Macrobii* (long-livers), a work devoted to longevity. He made these claims:

Nestor was an Argonaut, helped fight the centaurs, and participated in the hunt for the Calydonian Boar. He and his sons, Antilochus and Thrasymedes, fought on the side of the Achaeans in the Trojan war. Though Nestor was already old when the war began, he was noted for his bravery and speaking abilities. Lucian says that Nestor lived three centuries.

Tiresias, the blind seer of Thebes was alive for 600 years. In Greek mythology, Tiresias (Greek: Τειρεσίας, also transliterated as Teiresias) was a blind prophet of Thebes, famous for clairvoyance and for being transformed into a woman for seven years. He was the son of the shepherd Everes and the nymph Chariclo; Tiresias participated fully in seven generations at Thebes, beginning as advisor to Cadmus himself.

Abd el Aziz el Habachi (الا يزع لاز ح ب يش ع دب) was a unique case of long life mentioned by the founder of the Senussi Order, and also mentioned by the Moroccan scholar El Kettani (1888-1962) in his report "fahres el Fahares". According to sources he was born in 581 of the Hegira (1185 AD), and was a pupil of Ibn Hajar al-Asqalani (1372-1449) who claimed that Abd el Aziz was a 14th-generation descendant of the prophet Mohammed. He died in 1859 at the alleged age of 674 years.

Other sources say that he was present during the founding of the city of Cairo in 969, in the reign of El Moez El Fatimi (952-975). It was also claimed that he was near 900 years old when he died in 1859, according to Abd el Hamid Bik (died 1863) in "Aalam el Machareka Wa al Magariba" ("The Famous Men of the East and the West").

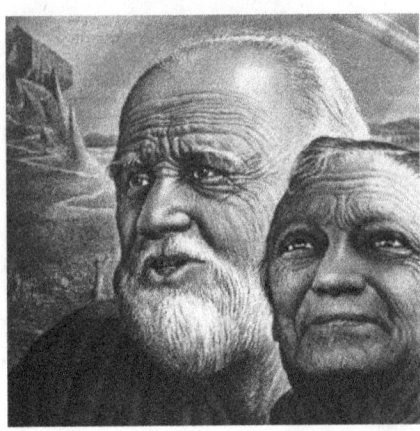

Long Lived Persons in the Bible

The Bible also has numerous persons in Genesis, Chapter 5 who lived much more than the normal life span.

If you believe in the Bible as a historical document or the word of God, then you should take the following statements in Genesis Chapter 5 seriously:

5:1 This is the book of the generations of Adam. In the day when God created man, He made him in the likeness of God.

2 He created them male and female, and He blessed them and named them Man in the day when they were created.

3 When Adam had lived one hundred and thirty years, he became the father of a son in his own likeness, according to his image, and named him Seth.

4 Then the days of Adam after he became the father of Seth were eight hundred years, and he had other sons and daughters.

5 So all the days that **Adam lived were nine hundred and thirty years**, and he died.

6 And Seth lived one hundred and five years, and became the father of Enosh.

7 Then Seth lived eight hundred and seven years after he became the father of Enosh, and he had other sons and daughters.

8 So **all the days of Seth were nine hundred and twelve years**, and he died.

9 And Enosh lived ninety years, and became the father of Kenan.

10 Then Enosh lived eight hundred and fifteen years after he became the father of Kenan, and he had other sons and daughters.

11 So **all the days of Enosh were nine hundred and five years**, and he died.

12 And Kenan lived seventy years, and became the father of Mahalalel.

13 Then Kenan lived eight hundred and forty years after he became the father of Mahalalel, and he had other sons and daughters.

14 So **all the days of Kenan were nine hundred and ten years**, and he died.

15 And Mahalalel lived sixty-five years, and became the father of Jared.

16 Then Mahalalel lived eight hundred and thirty years after he became the father of Jared, and he had other sons and daughters.

17 So **all the days of Mahalalel were eight hundred and ninety-five years**, and he died.

18 And Jared lived one hundred and sixty-two years, and became the father of Enoch.

19 Then Jared lived eight hundred years after he became the father of Enoch, and he had other sons and daughters.

20 So **all the days of Jared were nine hundred and sixty-two years**, and he died.

21 And Enoch lived sixty-five years, and became the father of Methuselah.

22 Then Enoch walked with God three hundred years after he became the father of Methuselah, and he had other sons and daughters.

23 So **all the days of Enoch were three hundred and sixty-five years**.

24 And Enoch walked with God; and he was not, for God took him.

25 And Methuselah lived one hundred and eighty-seven years, and became the father of Lamech.

26 Then Methuselah lived seven hundred and eighty-two years after he became the father of Lamech, and he had other sons and daughters.

27 So **all the days of Methuselah were nine hundred and sixty-nine years**, and he died.

28 And Lamech lived one hundred and eighty-two years, and became the father of a son.

29 Now he called his name Noah, saying, "This one shall give us rest from our work and from the toil of our hands arising from the ground which the LORD has cursed."

30 Then Lamech lived five hundred and ninety-five years after he became the father of Noah, and he had other sons and daughters.

31 So **all the days of Lamech were seven hundred and seventy-seven years**, and he died.

32 And **Noah was five hundred years old, and Noah became the father of Shem,** Ham, and Japheth.

Moses, the person who led the Israelites from Egypt is also stated in Deuteronomy to have lived to 120 years when he turned over the leadership of the Tribes to Jacob.

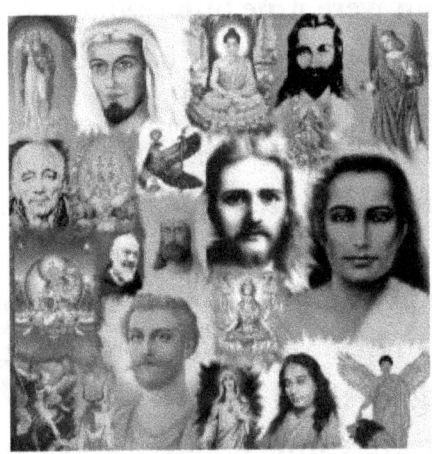

Ascended Master and Immortals

In this section we will read some incredible stores which strain credulity.

On the other hand, it's worth keeping an open mind since I've learned that almost anything is possible in this universe of ours.

One of the spiritual paths to physical immortality was brought to common knowledge in the West by the Theosophists and Indian yogis in the nineteenth century. It involves the teachings of Ascended Masters.

It is believed that Ascended Masters are individuals who were once embodied on Earth and learned the lessons of life in their incarnations. They gained mastery over the limitations of the matter planes, balanced at least 51% of their negative karma, and fulfilled their Dharma (Divine Plan). An Ascended Master has become God-like, and a source of unconditional love to all life, and through the Ascension has united with his or her own God Self, the "I AM" Presence.

It is claimed that they serve as the teachers of mankind from the realms of spirit, and that all people will eventually attain their Ascension and move forward in spiritual evolution beyond this planet.

According to these teachings, they remain attentive to the spiritual needs of humanity, and act to inspire and motivate it's spiritual growth. In many traditions and organizations, they are considered part of the Spiritual Hierarchy for Earth, and members of the Great Brotherhood of Light, also known as the Great White Lodge or Great White Brotherhood.

It is believed that if one can find ascended beings they will teach one how to become enlightened and physically immortal.

In the book "Breaking the Death Habit" Leonard Orr maintains that he met immortal Yogis in his travels in Asia. He says he met eight of them, male and female, and that three of them have been alive for over two thousand years.

He also says there are at least a few thousand immortals on the earth today and most live in the Himalayas.

I've read that 4,000 immortals meet at one festival in India every twelve years so there must be many more physical immortals. The majority live in China according to a well known Qi Gong teacher.

Many of them are not ascetics but have wives and children. This is important to know because it means you don't have to be an ascetic and live in a cave to become physically immortal.

He says that immortals enjoy their lives. "Abundant life is the Secret of Eternal life. Personal aliveness is the source of joy forever."

Babaji is one immortal who is supposed to be 9000 years old. Orr says the following about him in an interview:

Babaji systematically taught me the yoga of immortal yogis, and that is why I went to see him other than just to enjoy his presence. Because that body was 9000 years old and being in the presence of a 9000 year old person is unforgettable.

Babaji is also referenced in the book "Autobiography of a Yogi". Another immortal Orr met and discusses was Bhartriji:

It took Bhartriji 700 years to become totally enlightened; and to be able to manifest his thoughts at will in the physical universe. I wrote a book about him, and how he achieved physical immortality. When he was about 300 it was the height of his teaching career; and after that he surrendered to being a yogi. Babaji taught me that there are immortal yogis, but there aren't any immortal gurus. Bhartraji stopped talking about physical immortality; and just practices it except for once every 108 years he gives a public demonstration.

Other observations from Orr:

"The Siddha Ashram is kind of the fulfillment of what is popularized in the word Shambala. It's like an ashram which can be just some obscure village with all the members of the ashram are immortals who are 100's of years old, 1000's of year old. He evidently is a kind of missionary from that ashram to the West.

There are some immortals in the Philippines I've heard about. One guy is 300 and another 400. The guy who's 400 has a simple technique in that he just walks in the forest one day a week for 24 hours and communes with God. He doesn't eat or sleep for 24 hours, once a week. Very simple practice and he's been doing it for 400 years."

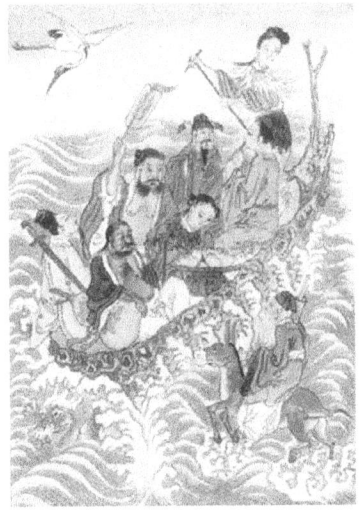

Taoist Immortals

Xian is a Chinese word for an enlightened person; translatable in English as:

"Spiritually immortal; transcendent; super-human; celestial being" (in Daoist/Taoist philosophy and cosmology.

The *Xian* archetype is described by Victor H. Mair:

They are immune to heat and cold, untouched by the elements, and can fly; mounting upward with a fluttering motion. They dwell apart from the chaotic world of man; subsist on air and dew, are not anxious like ordinary people, and have the smooth skin and innocent faces of children. The transcendent live an effortless existence that is best described as spontaneous. They recall the ancient Indian ascetics and holy men known as *ṛṣi,* who possessed similar traits.

The "*Yuan You*" ('Far-off Journey') poem describes a spiritual journey into the realms of Gods and immortals, frequently referring to Taoist myths and techniques.

> *My spirit darted forth and did not return to me,*
> *And my body, left tenantless, grew withered and lifeless.*
> *Then I looked into myself to strengthen my resolution,*
> *And sought to learn from where the primal spirit issues.*
> *In emptiness and silence I found serenity;*
> *In tranquil inaction I gained true satisfaction.*
> *I heard how once Red Pine had washed the world's dust off:*
> *I would model myself on the pattern he had left me.*
> *I honoured the wondrous powers of the Pure Ones,*
> *And those of past ages who had become immortals.*
> *They departed in the flux of change and vanished from men's sight,*
> *Leaving a famous name that endures after them.*

A recent book called the "Taoist Immortals" By Eva Wong discusses popular stories of famous Chinese immortals. Some of the stories have clues about how they became immortal.

One Taoist Immortal lived during the Shang dynasty (1766 B.C. to 1154 B. C.) was Peng-Tzu. The Chinese book of history lists him as having lived over 800 years.

Many Chinese immortals can be found in the book "A Gallery of Chinese Immortals".

Although there are different lists, the most famous are the Eight Taoist immortals which usually included the following persons:

Chung-li Ch'uan, the earliest in point of time, seems to have been chiefly responsible for the formation of the group. Tradition makes him a Han general, but there is no real evidence to show that he was an historical personage; and, considering his popular renown, he has but few striking exploits to his credit. His birth was accompanied by strange phenomena, and several physical peculiarities are recorded. All his life he was a wanderer.

He was converted to Tao by an aged man whom he met in a remote village. Towards the end of his career he fell in with the Taoist adept T'ao Hung-ching, and received from him "a pinch of the Great Monad" (a mysterious cosmic entity existing before the evolution of material things), a fire-charm, and some spiritual elixir. Artists depict him as a fat, bearded old man, scantily clad, and carrying a feathered fan with fly-whisk attached, or sometimes a two edged sword.

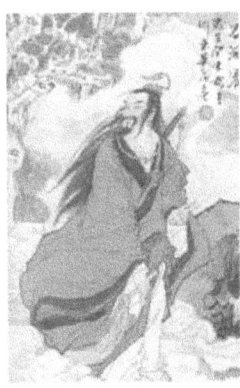

Chang Kuo was a hermit whose origin is unknown. It was his custom to ride a white donkey, on which he could cover immense distances in a single day. When he stopped to rest, he would fold the animal up like paper, and put it away in his cap- box. Then, when he was ready to start again, he sprayed water over it from his mouth, and changed it back into a donkey. He is said to have been invited to Court by more than one of the early T'ang emperors, but did not respond until the reign of Ming Huang, who treated him with great respect.

On receiving another summons, however, he immediately lay down and died. He was buried in the usual way by his disciples, but subsequently, when the coffin was

opened, it was found to be quite empty. Pictures of Chang Kuo show him seated on his donkey and holding a musical instrument called a fish-drum, which looks like a golf-bag with two clubs (really castanets) protruding from it. Lu Yen (or familiarly, Lu Tung-pin), also of the T'ang dynasty, is probably the most popular member of the group. Though he is said to have failed twice for the doctor's degree, he is widely worshipped as a patron saint of literature. He became the pupil of an old Taoist encountered by chance, who was no other than Chung-li Ch'uan. During a period of probation

before he became a Hsien, he had to undergo a series of ten ordeals. The last of these was the hostile approach of a host of demons in terrifying shapes, which left him completely undismayed. Once he fell asleep while a meal of yellow millet was cooking, and dreamt of events extending over the best part of a lifetime; yet on awaking he found the millet still uncooked.

His emblem is the magic two edged sword which conferred the gift of invisibility, and enabled him to overcome evil spirits.

Ts'ao Kuo-chiu is said, on dubious authority, to have been the younger brother of a Sung empress in the eleventh century, "a handsome youth of peaceful disposition". One day, in the course of their wanderings, Chung-li Ch'uan and Lu Tung-pin came to his dwelling-place, and asked to be told the object of his spiritual meditations. "Tao alone," he replied, "is the object which I have in view."—"And where is Tao?" [sic] asked the two hsien. Kuo-chiu pointed up to heaven.--"Where then is heaven?"--Kuo-chiu pointed to his heart. Chung-li Ch'uan smiled and said: "The heart is one with heaven, and heaven is one with Tao? Nay, then you have a true understanding of the essential constitution of

things." And accordingly they admitted him to the company of immortals.

Ts'ao Kuo-chiu is usually represented as a bearded grandee in Court attire. His distinctive attribute is, somewhat incongruously, a pair of clapper castanets.

Li T'ieh-kuai, that is, "Li with the Iron Staff", is depicted as a lame and repulsive-looking beggar, though originally he was a handsome, well-built man. This is how the transformation came about. When he was setting off to meet Lao Tzu on one of the sacred mountains, he told a disciple that only the spiritual part of him was making the journey, while his body would remain behind. If the spirit should not return within seven days, the body might be burnt. Now, the disciple was anxious to visit his sick brother, so he left on the sixth day, after burning the body. Consequently, when the Master's spirit returned on the following day, it had nowhere to go, until at last it entered and re-animated the corpse of a beggar who had died of starvation. Thereafter Li T'ieh-kuai walked the earth in the guise of a cripple, clad in rags and tatters.

In pictures he is seen hobbling along with the aid of a staff. Out of a bottle-gourd in his hand there rises a mysterious vapor, in which appears an emblem of his spiritual self.

Han Hsiang Tzu was a nephew of the great T'ang poet Han Yu. At birth he had all the marks of a future hsien. Of an eccentric disposition, he hated all the pomps and vanities of the world, and delighted in stillness and obscurity. His mind was absorbed in the art of alchemy and the pursuit of "the elixir". When urged by his uncle to apply himself to study, he replied: "The object of my study is different from yours." He was instructed by Chung-li Ch'uan and Lu Tung-pin in their system of Tao, and followed them on their wanderings. Coming to a peach-tree, he climbed up to pluck the fruit of immortality, but was thrown to the ground by the snapping of a branch and was killed. At the very same moment he was transfigured and became a hsien. Afterwards, in the guise of a Taoist priest, he tried to convert his uncle, who was a strong confucianist, and succeeded at least in convincing him

that he was no charlatan. His attribute is a flute, besides which he is often to be seen with a pair of long castanets and an alchemist's crucible.

Lan Ts'ai-ho is portrayed as a ragged, unkempt, good-looking youth, sometimes even as a girl. All accounts of this hsien are purely legendary, but he is said to have gone about with one foot bare, singing crazy songs which he improvised as he went along. In summer he stuffed his gown with cotton-wool, while in winter he would sleep in the snow, with vapour rising from his body like steam. When drunk, he used to sing and caper, and was followed by crowds of people who did not know what to make of his antics. The cash which he received as alms he would thread on a string and trail behind him as he walked. If any were lost, he would pay no heed. He used to give his money to the poor, or spend it in wine-taverns. It was from a wine-tavern that he eventually soared up to the sky on the back of a crane. This strange being is generally shown with a basket full of flowers and plants associated with longevity, such as chrysanthemums, plum-blossoms, sprigs of pine and bamboo, etc.

Ho Hsien Ku is the only undoubted female hsien belonging to the group. At the age of fourteen or fifteen she dreamt that she was visited by a divinity who advised her to eat powdered mica in order to etherealize her body. She also met a stranger who gave her a peach, and on returning home she found that she had been absent not for one day, as she had supposed, but for a whole month; yet she was not one whit the worse for going all that time without food. Having made a vow of chastity, she withdrew into the mountains, where she would flit to and fro like a bird.

Towards the beginning of the eighth century she is said to have ascended on high in broad daylight. Ho Hsien Ku's special emblem is a bamboo ladle, for which the following explanation is given: she had a stepmother who treated her harshly and kept her toiling all day long over menial domestic duties. Despite this, she behaved with such exemplary patience the Lu Tung-pin was moved to come and rescue her from her miserable drudgery. He found her busy in the kitchen, and as he bore her upwards the ladle she was using still remained in her hand.

Chapter Summary

In this chapter my objective was to present the reader with enough information to overwhelm their previous beliefs about how long a person can live.

I think I've presented a enough evidence here about extraordinary longevity to convince most people that the possibility exists.

But there is another issue to confront too:

When I give my workshops and lectures I usually ask the audience "How old would you like to live and why?"

Most people pick an age of seventy or eighty and their why their answer is very revealing. Most of them say they don't want to live to an age where they will be sick, immobile, or infirm.

When you review the evidence of very long lived people you will see that all of the supercentenarians are not only healthy, but very physically active.

In fact, a high level of physical activity into extreme old age is one of the secrets of living to 150 years or beyond.

Once a person understands that a very long life is really possible, then the next question is does this person have a purpose in their life to keep living.

We will cover life purpose in the next chapter.

3.0 Defining Your Purpose in Life

The second principle of personal longevity is having a life purpose or mission in life.

When I was designing these principles I realized that if each of us doesn't have a purpose in living— then what is the point?

Therefore an early step in the extended longevity process is to define why we are here on earth and what are we living for?

Life Without a Purpose:

The Dalai Lama sums up the lack of purpose in many of our lives today:

- *We have more conveniences, but less time.*
- *We have more degrees, but less sense more knowledge but less judgment. More experts, but more problems. More medicines, but less healthiness.*
- *We have been all the way to the moon and back but have trouble crossing the street to meet the new neighbor.*
- *We build more computers to hold more information that produce more copies than ever before, but have less communication.*
- *We have become long on quantity, but short on quality. These are the times of fast foods but weak digestion. It is a time when there is much in the window but nothing in the room.*

Not knowing one's purpose is one of the biggest problems in life around the world today.

Not everyone can be a gifted composer or scientist—yet we all have a true uniqueness as our gift from God.

Each of us has at least one unique thing to contribute to this world-ourselves.

Maybe your purpose in life it to be a friend to others, or to just provide some comfort to a person in need.

Our life purpose doesn't have to be big—it just has to be something from deep in our soul that satisfies our reason for incarnating in this life.

How I know my Soul's Purpose?

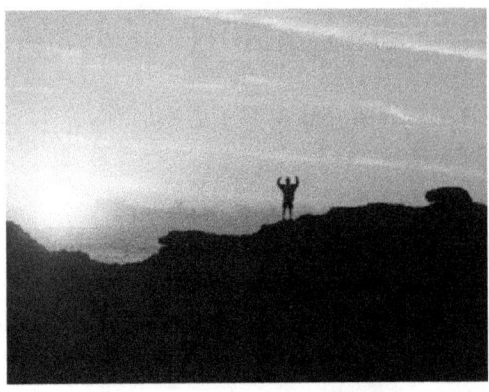

I have been blessed with many wonderful experiences in my life.

The first blessing in my life was that I remember before I was born, my gestation, and my birth.

I remember being part of a larger super consciousness in another realm of the spirit. That I felt the need to return to the earth to accomplish a new mission.

Other similar consciousnesses around me told me that I had already done a lot of work on the earth and didn't need to go back. My decision was firm though—I knew this incarnation needed to be accomplished and I was determined to do it.

I broke off a portion of my spirit into a smaller package and came down to the earth to choose a mother and father.

My recollection is that my goal in choosing parents was to find a pair of well-educated parents who would be well grounded in life-thus raising me to be well grounded.

There were several candidate couples in upstate New York. I choose a candidate and came closer to my new mother to be. When I got close I was drawn inside of her womb and my spirit became attached to the embryo growing there.

At one point the cord was choking me so I had to turn around to get it from around my neck.

I remember growing in my mom's womb—then it became too small and I felt compressed. Eventually it became so tight that my mom's water broke and I started being forced out.

I was a breach birth and came out feet first. The compression pain was great when I passed through my mom's birth canal/

After I was born I recall breathing on my own. Then the doctor held me up and hit my butt—I spasmed and took in a great breath of air—which felt like fire in my lungs. His overly powerful slap of my bottom also caused congestion in my lungs so I was placed in an iron lung for a few hours.

At the age of two years old I was sitting in my living room watching an old boxy black and white TV— then I remember that I was waking up from some type of dream I'd been living for the last couple of years. That I knew I was alive and here to accomplish my mission on earth!

Much of my teenage years were consumed with curiosity about the spiritual and paranormal. Without much information available from my parents and friends I found books to read which satisfied my thirst for knowledge.

Throughout my childhood I still knew that I had an important purpose in life—but wasn't sure what it was.

Later in my teens I was drawn to read books on the paranormal, try ESP experiments read lots of Science Fiction.

In college I met a spiritual Mentor named Sam Lentine who taught me how to meditate, and to take in energy through my crown chakra.

In parallel with a traditional business career for thirty years, I had many spiritual and paranormal experiences. (Which I've covered in some of my other books)

In 2008 I just felt it was time to start writing on what I could research and what I knew about different spiritual and paranormal subjects.

Now in early 2013 I know that the last five years I was building a foundation of knowledge, books, videos, and other materials to prepare me for my real life's work.

My real life's work turns out to be that of a Spiritual Teacher and counselor on long term health and extreme longevity.

How do I know this? It's not an analytical answer but a spiritual one—that I now feel I'm in spiritual alignment with my life's purpose.

This alignment makes me excited about the future, and I can't wait to implement my training program.

My alignment with my spirit's goals energizes me and just gives me a deep "knowing" that I'm on the right track.

It's hard to express, but I just know I was meant to be on this path.

Everything I've learned and experienced up until this point in life is part of this path.

My point in relating the above story was to show how I became certain of my life's purpose. Hopefully you will have a similar awakening.

Having these types of feelings about your life is how you know you have found your life's calling. You don't need to go through all of the events of my life to find your Soul's Purpose.

By introspection and some of the exercises offered later in this chapter you can find what that purpose really is.

Who you Really are:

A good starting point on defining your Soul's Purpose is to determine who you really are. You should ask questions of your family and friends to help you better grasp why you are here:

What are you reflecting back to yourself by not allowing yourself to see or know your soul's purpose? Who supports you in living your soul's purpose and who does not support you?

Who of all of your friends would be there for you to support you in discovering your soul's purpose and following through with you on bringing it to the surface?

Ask each family member, young or old; what do they think is your soul's purpose?

Write down each person's answer, without comment or judgment. Also, ask each personal friend or co-worker what they think is your soul's purpose. This will help you in discovering your soul's purpose.

Once you realize what your soul's purpose is – you will stop wasting your time by distracting yourself from what you really aught to be doing.-Deborah Skye King

Many cases of depression and listlessness are the result of not knowing what you are meant to do on this earth in this lifetime.

The joy and happiness you experience in life are in many ways linked to how well you are working towards your life's path or purpose.

Did you ever see a depressed person who was doing their real life's work? Or a person energized about their work if they saw no purpose to it?

Your Mission in Life:

Why is it important to have a mission in life? Here are some quotes from the Bible that may help answer that question:

It is God himself who has made us what we are and given us new lives from Christ Jesus; and long ages ago he planned that we should spend these lives in helping others. Ephesians 2:10

I glorified you on earth by completing down to the last detail what you assigned me to do. John 17:4 You were put on earth to make a contribution.

You weren't created just to consume resources—to eat, breathe, and take up space. God designed you to make a difference with your life. While many best-selling books offer advice on how to "get" the most out of life, that's not the reason God made you. You were created to add to life on earth, not just

take from it. God wants you to give something back. This is God's fourth purpose for your life, and it is called your "ministry," or service. The Bible gives us the details. You were created to serve God.

- The Purpose Driven Life: What on Earth Am I Here For? By Rick Warren

Building a Life Purpose:

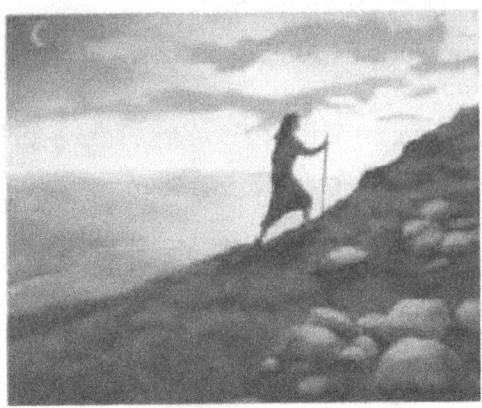

What is Purpose?

Ancient writers wrote a lot about this topic. An ancient Tibetan text states that a life purpose is "*for the benefit of self and for the benefit of others.*"

Below are four quotations relevant to the issue of life purpose that we give to ILCT participants, asking them to reflect on what the quotes mean to them. These four seem to be particularly meaningful quotations that move students toward introspective thinking about the importance of life purpose and the variety of ways to describe it.

When we are motivated by goals that have deep meaning, by dreams that need completion, by pure love that needs expressing, then we truly live life.

We can define "purpose" in several ways. For one, when we know our purpose, we have an anchor— a device of the mind to provide some stability, to keep from tossing us to and fro, from inflicting constant seasickness on us. Or we can think of our purpose as being a master nautical chart marking shoals and rocks, sandbars and derelicts, something to guide us and keep us on course. Perhaps the most profound thing we can say about being "on purpose" is that when that is our status, our condition, and our comfort, we find our lives have meaning, and when we are "off purpose," we are confused about meanings and motives.

The first principle of ethical power is Purpose By purpose, I mean your objective or intention—

something toward which you are always striving. Purpose is something bigger. It is the picture you have of yourself— the kind of person you want to be or the kind of life you want to lead.

A purpose is more ongoing and gives meaning to our lives. When people have a purpose in

life, they enjoy everything they do more! People go on chasing goals to prove something that doesn't have to be proved: that they're already worthwhile.

There are a variety of techniques we can use to zero in on our true life purpose.

Here are some exercises to help you create a life purpose statement:

(From Becoming a Professional Life Coach)

1. List the top ten things you love to do or have always done and loved. Name several things you have consistently made part of your life, regardless of the circumstances. Examples might include networking with like-minded people, your faith or spirituality, your creativity at work, your heartfelt communications, or your ability to take action under pressure.
2. Identify the characteristics of the context or environment that support your list from Step 1. List the qualities of people you want and need to be around to accomplish your top ten. Draw a series of concentric circles on a blank piece of paper, and write "ME" in the center circle. Each circle represents a group of people who are important to you. Put the names of those closest to you, who affect your life most, in the circle next to you. Then continue to draw your circles outward: family, friends, work colleagues, professional groups, community, and so on. In each circle, write a few words that describe the qualities this group must embody to support you in just the way you need and want. Then identify other resources that are essential to you: peacefulness, time in nature, other creative people, and so on. Ask yourself, "What are the essential supporting features of the world I want to live in so that I can be at my best?"
3. Using the phrases you generated in Step 2, write one to two sentences that express your vision of the world you want to live in. This is the path of least resistance for you, the world you flourish in and want to create for yourself through purpose-full action. Crystallize the essence of your vision.

For example, "My vision is that all people of the world will be able to live their lives by choice— in a way that matters to them." This vision expresses the fact that choice is essential for the writer.

Once we have a long term purpose then extended longevity (physical immortality) becomes an important goal to strive for.

Setting Goals

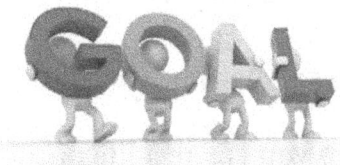

Once you have developed your life purpose it's time to set goals to accomplish it.

Only 3% of the world's population set goals—and they accomplish more than the other 97% combined.

Dr. John F. Dimartini describes the process of goal setting:

- Goals are to be of a realistic nature.
- Goals are to be believable to you and achievable.
- Goals are to be specific, the more detail the better.
- Goals are to be harmonious with your higher values. They should be created with what you already know or are interested in.
- Goals are to be prioritized; having a list of what you desire creates a stronger foundation from which to work.
- Goals are to be given completion and achievement dates. This way you can have markers for what is being created and what you need to do in order to complete a goal.

Setting a Course of Action:

1. Begin the day with an open mind toward what you desire to create in the moment
2. Write down any challenges you think you may encounter
3. Set up a plan for how you will accomplish your goals

4. If any challenges occur, remember to have a marker, something that will show you that you have arrived at your predetermined destination, so you will know you have accomplished what you have set out to.

Living in Awareness

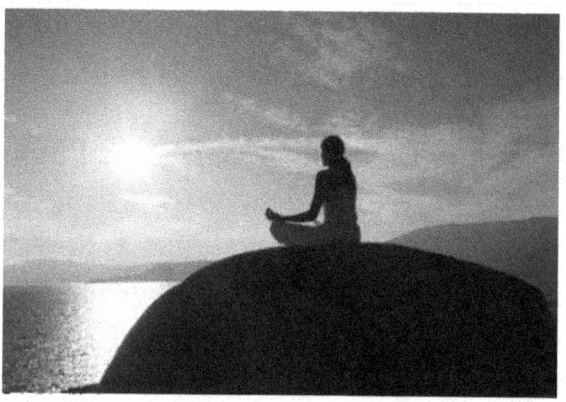

We should learn to bring awareness from the Soul to everything we do. This allows us to be authentic—to know our real selves.

When we do this we are more in touch with our Soul's needs and purpose in life.

Do you give thanks for everything you do?

How about when you are brushing your teeth in the morning—do you give thanks for that action? Do you notice the pleasure you have in each bite of food you take?

Do you think about the words you are saying to others and their effect on them and you?

What about thanks for your every breath—without continuous breathing you wouldn't last very long.

Living in awareness is all about clearly seeing and experiencing our environment from minute to minute—and living in the present.

Being aware at this level helps you to understand if you are doing something worthwhile or living in emptiness.

This level of awareness will also help you live in the heart to experience unconditional love too.

Life Purpose Summary:

Finding your purpose and goals in life is not a one-time thing. Although your true purpose should remain constant, the goals that are most important to you will change throughout your life.

This is since we go through different phases of life, and our goals to implement our soul's purpose may change in those different stages of life.

Good luck and many blessings on finding your Soul's Purpose and achieving it in this life!

Now that you know your purpose in life another challenge is your belief that you can live a long time. This issue is called by various names:

- Removing the Death Urge
- Enabling your Life Urge
- Having a Positive Outlook on life

In the next chapter we will review the psychology of believing you really can live a long time.

4.0 Enabling Your Life Urge

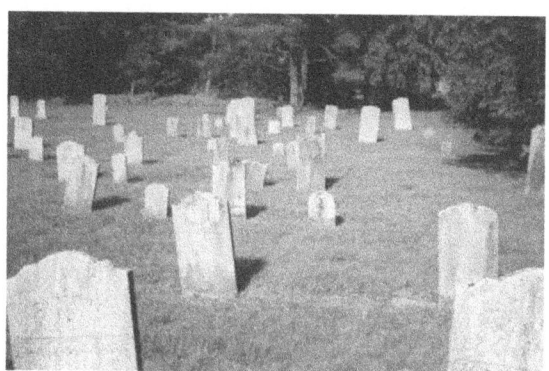

The Third Principle of personal longevity is about changing the subconscious programming we all learn from birth in our society.

This programming is that we are expected to go through certain stages in life and then die. An example from my life:

I had a paper route when I was eleven years old and one of my customers was an old couple in their eighties—family friends named the Burrus.

They were very healthy until the man died one day—I don't know from what. After that his wife got thinner and thinner each week that I saw her until she just died after six more months because she had no more will to live.

She had decided it was her time to die.

How many of us have known persons like this who just gave up and quit?

You have to want to live and long time and know that you can do it to make it possible in your life.

We can change our programming to know deep down that we are able to live much longer and have more fulfilling lives than we ever thought possible.

Leonard Orr:

Much of the wisdom on the life urge is from the teachings of Leonard Orr. Leonard is an unconventional thinker of the 1960s and 1970s.

He started the re-birthing movement in San Francisco during the 1960's New Age era in San

Francisco. He also wrote a book called "Breaking the Death Habit" which is now out of print but can be obtained at my website http://mkettingtonbooks.com

In this book he says that he met many immortals in India and the Himalayas who were all at least 300 years old or more.

He learned a lot of his knowledge from an ascended master "Babaji" who has been around for thousands of years.

He says that disciples first need to work on developing a philosophy of physical immortality.

Leonard says: "The physiology of physical immortality is based on inner awareness of our energy body. One must learn how to clean and balance the energy body on a daily basis with earth, air, water, and fire.

Second you need to unravel the "Death Urge" which is built into all family traditions through the psychology of physical immortality. By this Leonard means the expectation built into almost everyone's subconscious that we will all live an average life span, and then die.

Here are some of the death urges built into our subconscious which we learn growing up in our civilization:

The belief that we will physically slow down starting in our thirties, become much less mobile in our sixties and bedridden in our eighties

The image we project on older people that they aren't as attractive or healthy as younger people— this image affects them too

Advertising to start planning for your own funeral

Retirement Planning only looking at a timeframe of living into your eighties—because you will not need any money after that Social Security and Medicare—we will not be able to take care of ourselves when we retire

The belief that the mind will lose its memory and ability to think clearly as it ages That old people are ugly

That there will be nothing interesting to do after kids move away and we retire from our job That old people need to make space in society for the young

Medical care being reduced for old people, and sometimes withheld—because they will die anyway

The third step is the mastery of the physical body. This can be accomplished by certain breathing exercises and practices.

The final step is where spiritual purification exercises come in.

We recommend people start by saying the following to themselves every day:

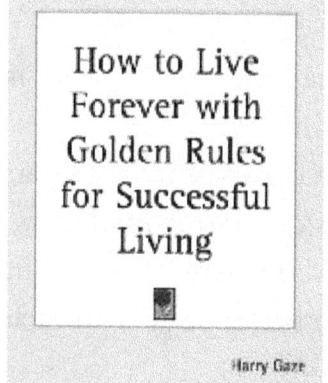

"My life urges are strong, in control, and keep me continuously alive and in perfect robust health.

The following book by Harry Gaze in an excellent source of re-programing and positive thinking to help us change our programming about how long we believe we can live.

Golden Rules to Live Forever

Harry Gaze was a Philosopher and Teacher back in the early 20th Century. He was a teacher and lecturer in practical Metaphysics, New Thought, and Divine Science. He began his lecture work as early as 1898 and published numerous books on Metaphysics.

His book titled "How to Live Forever with Golden Rules for Successful Living" is very relevant to our study of physical immortality, and was first published in 1905. (He also wrote an earlier work on the subject in 1904 titled "How to Live Forever, The Science and Practice").

Like some other writers on the subject of unlimited longevity he believed that growing old and the body decaying was not inevitable! His belief was that the power of the spirit and thought on the body could keep one young forever.

Harry believed in several principles which guided his thinking:

The body literally and completely returns to dust in less than one year, and during this period, a new body is constructed molecule by molecule.

Conscious cooperation with this change is the secret to eternal youth.

Old age and somatic death are brought about by conditions which can be effectually prevented. He had a set of Golden Rules for Eternal Youth which are reproduced here:

1. *Golden Rule for Eternal Youth Number One*: Realize there is one divine life in which you live, move, and have your being.
2. *Golden Rule for Eternal Youth Number Two*: Realize that as a Son of God you are heir to God's immortality here and now; claim your birthright.
3. *Golden Rule for Eternal Youth Number Three*: Realize that your body is a template of the Holy Spirit.
4. *Golden Rule for Eternal Youth Number Four*: Deeply realize that your body is an expression of your mind, and attune yourself to infinite spirit.
5. *Golden Rule for Eternal Youth Number Five*: Realize that by virtue of molecular renewal, which is constantly in operation, your body is constantly made new.
6. *Golden Rule for Eternal Youth Number Six*: Keep in mind that nature's constant renewal of the body gives the opportunity of building a better body with each succeeding renewal.
7. *Golden Rule for Eternal Youth Number Seven*: Practice rhythmical breathing and freely use your diaphragm, the organ that is the muscular floor of your upper internal organs, and the ceiling of your lower organs.
8. *Golden Rule for Eternal Youth Number Eight*: Realize that eternal youth is harmony and positive cooperation with the upward law of continuous growth and the law of attraction.
9. *Golden Rule for Eternal Youth Number Nine*: Realize that the secret of eternal youth is cooperation with God in creative, individual, volitional evolution.
10. *Golden Rule for Eternal Youth Number Ten*: Practice faithfully the daily affirmations for Eternal Youth, doing them in a regular, cumulative sequence.

11. *Golden Rule for Eternal Youth Number Eleven:* Practice concentrative exercises daily, and develop control of attention and thought selectivity. Also do meditative exercises and the Silence.

(Note the focus on meditation in Rule Eleven. This was a very unusual term to use one hundred years ago and indicates some familiarity with knowledge from the East.)

12. *Golden Rule for Eternal Youth Number Twelve:* Realize the oneness of your inner Christ life with God, thinking of God as an Infinite Life, Infinite Power, Infinite Health, Infinite Youth, Infinite Peace, Infinite Joy.

Rule number 10 mentions the daily affirmations for Eternal Youth. These are listed below too. Mr. Gaze recommends practicing one daily for the whole month, then starting over again:

- Adaptation: Whenever essential, I adapt myself readily to more perfect change.
- Adjustment: I give myself freely to wise, spiritual, mental, and physical adjustment.
- Beauty: I realize that the beauty of enduring youth is as deep as the innermost recesses of the soul.
- Buoyancy: In every thought, nerve, and muscle I express the perfect buoyancy of joyous youth.
- Confidence: I cheerfully react to all conditions with the boundless confidence of youth.
- Courage: I increasingly attain the natural courage of strong and vital youth.
- Creativeness: The Divine Spirit, everywhere, and in and through me, inspires me with keen creativeness.
- Daring: I blend the pure daring of youth with the wisdom of growth and experience.
- Elasticity: My sense of freedom and flexibility of mind find its correspondence in bodily elasticity.
- Energy: My whole being is vitally energized with the radiant life of the Divine Spirit.
- Flexibility: I joyously affirm the quality of flexibility in every cell, muscle and artery of my being.
- Freshness: Bathing in the commonness of pure spirit, I am fresh as the dawn of day.

- Gracefulness: By wise exercise, relaxation, visualization and nourishment, I maintain the gracefulness of youth.
- Happiness: I realize that the true spring of happiness is within me.
- Initiative: The spirit of initiative and wise adventure freely motivates and activates me.
- Joy: The joy of eternal youth is my daily light and inspiration.
- Loveliness: The loveliness of ever-renewing youth is the expression of loving and lovable qualities.
- Newness: Every day and every moment, my body is being made new in every cell, molecule and atom.
- Optimism: I look joyously forward with the spirit of youthful optimism.
- Progressiveness: I am a progressive conscious, purposeful and individual factor in my evolution.
- Purity: I see life with the eyes of childlike purity blended with power and poise.
- Radiance: I am radiant with the light, life and love of infinite wisdom.
- Receptivity: Knowing that l am a child of God, l am at all times receptive to the highest inspiration.
- Rejuvenation: I am devoted and consecrated to all habits that rejuvenate and heal.
- Renewal: I am an ever-renewing and ever-unfolding expression of infinite life.
- Responsiveness: As the years unfold, I maintain my full, free responsiveness to the best in life.
- Unfoldment: I am open, receptive and responsive to new growth and unfoldments.
- Versatility: I joyously express the creative spirit in me in the versatility that unites youth with experience.
- Vitality: I think, speak, breathe, exercise, relax and nourish my mind and body for increasing vitality.
- Youth: I realize that the fountain of Eternal Youth, like the Kingdom of God, is here and now, within me.
- Zest: My thought, speech and action are all radiantly animated with youthful zest for living.

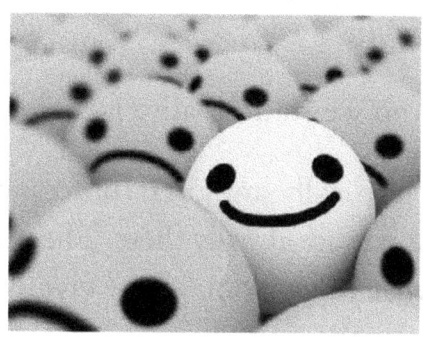

A Positive Outlook on Life

How does a positive outlook on life increase your life span?

Optimism and a positive outlook increases our vitality and spiritual connections.

If you are positive you have a better chance of extracting yourself from an unhealthful or dangerous situation.

An article extract from an M.D. reinforces the importance of a positive outlook:

"Optimism is necessary for good health," says Charles L. Raison, MD, a psychiatrist and director of the behavioral immunology clinic at Emory University School of Medicine in Atlanta. "There's growing evidence that, for many medical illnesses, stress and a negative mental state -- pessimism, feeling overwhelmed, being burnt out -- has a negative effect on immunity, which is especially important in rheumatoid arthritis."

Indeed, your brain can create all sorts of tailor-made prescriptions to nurture your body. Raison says these include endorphins -- the natural painkillers; gamma globulin, which fortifies your immune system; and interferon, which helps combat infections, viruses, even cancer.

When depression sets in, we're less likely to take care of ourselves, which means the brain doesn't get prompted to produce those great natural remedies, Raison says. We don't exercise, because we don't have much energy. We don't eat right. We lose sleep -- or we sleep too much.

Visualizing your Immortal Future

Here is an exercise to help you see yourself alive far into the future...

The key to visualizing your physically immortal future is not to imagine that you will get there but to imagine that you are already there. The more vividly you can imagine being immortal now and what you are doing very vividly, the more this changes the probability of your future to make it so.

Here is an excellent exercise to help you visualize yourself in health and happiness in your own immortal future:

Relax for 5-10 minutes.

Choose a happy scene of family, friends, or profession or activities that you want to visualize.

We are going to picture the scene you have chosen at different ages. These ages will be 100, 200, and 500 years old. As you visualize you will be in that scene. You make it real. You will put energy and will into it to make it happen.

You are now 100 years old. You are in the scene. People and scenery are around you. You can feel the temperature; the light in the sky or ceiling. You also smell the scene and you see everything vividly. You can look around and see details such as trees or on buildings or walls, etc.

Your body feels healthy and you can tell you are youthful. Your solid belief in your own immortality has been paying off for a while now.

You are now 200 years old and it's the 23rd century. (Your lifestyle may have changed to something which is an earlier period in a place where change is slower). Again, see your surroundings very vividly in a scene you enjoy. Feel all five senses.

- What do you see?
- What do you hear?
- What do you smell?
- What do you taste?
- What do you feel?

You are now 500 years old and it's the 25th century. You may have travelled out into the solar system or to a planet around another star. Life goes on and you are in a community of other immortals who have similar interests to you.

Maybe you are getting educated for a new profession, or maybe you are an artist in a mode you never tried before. You have probably learned to teleport yourself by this time and live totally in the now. Look around you to see what's there. You feel very strong and healthy as you usually do, and you have now been healthy and physically stable for centuries.

Keep doing this imagery consistently every day for a few minutes until you start to feel solidity and that the events will happen. This is when you now that your will and energy have created the future.

You might want to record this visualization on tape to play back to yourself. Your own voice is the most powerful voice you can hear.

Chapter Summary

At this point in your reading you should know that a very long life is possible, have some idea of your life purpose, and have an understanding of the beliefs that you can do it yourself.

In the next chapter we will get to the key topic of our individual spiritual connections and how that helps improve our long term health.

5.0 The Importance of a Spiritual Connection

The fourth principle of personal longevity is that we all need a spiritual connection in our lives.

It doesn't matter what religion or practices you believe in. What matters is the connection of the core of your being to the eternal spirit.

This can be done through deep prayers, meditation, or just walking in the woods and communing with nature.

Many people don't believe that we even have an eternal spirit at the core of our being. Therefore I think it's important to address that issue.

Astrophysics and relativity theory provide some interesting insights into the very probable scenario that another level of existence does exist which is a timeless and space less realm which is what all the mystics tell us is the realm of the spirit.

The Reality of Stillness

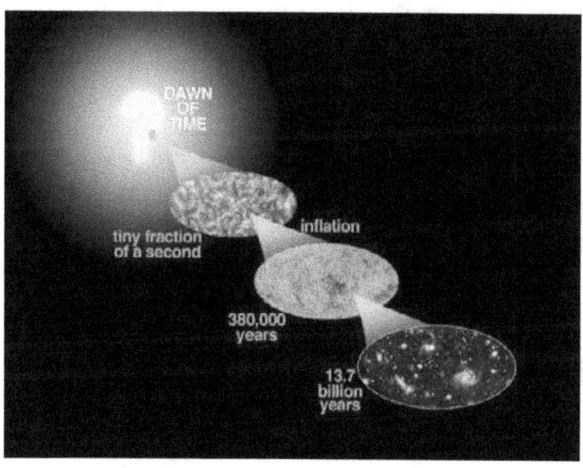

The growth of the Universe

Most people believe that God was the initial creative force which started the Universe.

Physicists and Astronomers all agree that the Universe we know was created from nothing and inflated in a huge explosion called the "Big Bang". As it inflated time and space as we know them came into existence.

When you study Einstein's Relativistic physics you being to understand that time and space are inextricably linked. You can't have one without the other.

Given our understanding of physics, we know that time and space didn't exist before the Big Bang. The state of things before creation then was "No Time & No Space".

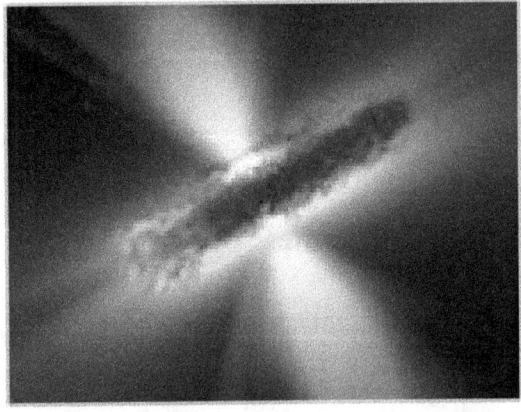

A notional picture of a black hole

Another subject of great interest to astrophysicists is what are called "Black Holes". Black Holes are a result of Einstein's equations and astronomers have verified their existence in the last few decades.

Black Holes are stars which due to their own mass have collapsed down to an infinitely small point and where time stops. Scientists do not understand where all that mass goes.

Hmm…. A Black Hole seems to be another example of part of reality that exists without time and space.

In Quantum Physics, time is also viewed differently than we perceive it on a daily basis. Here is a quote from a Physics website explaining this view:

The upshot is that, on the microscopic level, there is no direction to time -- and this is even more spectacularly true in quantum physics than in classical physics. In the microscopic domain, everything just exists in a kind of nebulous, atemporal continuum. Then, every once in a while, something becomes observable, and enters the one-dimensional time continuum. The arrow of time does not exist in the universe as a whole. It only exists in individual subjective views of the universe!

I think it is fair to say that the place of stillness where time and space don't exist is part of our reality.

Therefore, it shouldn't be considered too strange that our immortal spirit is part of and one with that stillness.

Finding Stillness in Major Religions

Christianity is the largest religion in the world, and one I know pretty well since I was raised in Methodist and Presbyterian churches growing up. I also attended multiple churches as an adult and participated in Bible study groups for a number of years.

Prayer is the key to stillness as a Christian. There are many books on Prayer and Prayer techniques. One needs to focus on spirit and becoming one with the spirit to move towards a state of stillness as a Christian.

The fact that so many of the long lived persons recorded in this book lived in Christian cultures probably indicates that being a devoted Christian can help you "live in the spirit" as much as many other spiritual techniques.

I'm not as familiar with Judaism and Islam, but the same approach applies in doing prayers in those religions.

The key to Prayer in your religion or spiritual approach is that you must learn to focus on the spirit of God which is inside you; and is the core of your being. That spirit exists in eternal peace; outside of time and space.

Once you learn to focus on that spirit in your prayer you will be able to bring that peace and stillness into your physical body to calm it and provide more health.

Biblical Quotes Relating to Stillness and the Spirit

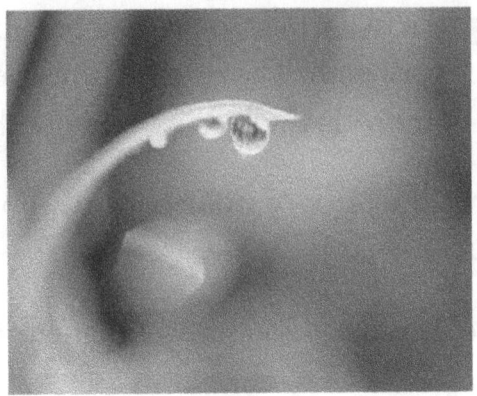

Here are a number of Biblical quotes which relate to the power of the spirit and the state of stillness (peace) I've described above.

> You will experience God's peace which is far more wonderful than the human mind can understand. His peace will keep your thoughts and your hearts quiet and at rest as you trust in Jesus Christ. (Philippians 4:7 LB)

> He will keep in perfect peace all those who trust in him, whose thoughts turn often to the Lord. (Isaiah 26:3 LB)

> The work of righteousness shall be peace; and the effect of righteousness, quietness and assurance forever. (Isaiah 32:17 KJV)

> "You shall receive power when the Holy Spirit has come upon you; and you shall be my witnesses both in Jerusalem, and in all Judea and Samaria, and even to the remotest part of the Earth. (Acts 1:8 NASB)

> For by one Spirit are we all baptized into one body (1 Corinthians 12:13 KJV)

> I will ask the Father and he will give you another Comforter, and he will never leave you. He is the Holy Spirit. The spirit who leads into all truth. The world at large cannot receive him; for it isn't looking for him and doesn't recognize him. But you do, for he lives with you now, and some day shall be in you. (John 14:16,17 LB)

> Do you not know that you are a temple of God and that the spirit of God dwells within you? (1 Corinthians 3:16 NASB)

There are many more quotes about the spirit of God, but the key is that they all relate to that core of God's spirit inside us all.

Spiritual Growth Practices

This chapter is intended as a guide to some of the spiritual practices which can be used to make your physical body healthier and younger.

It is not an exclusive list since I'm sure there are many paths which all go to enlightenment; with immortality as a side benefit.

In fact, the goal of spiritual growth should be enlightenment—not immortality. However, since immortality is the subject of this book I'm really focusing on a side effect of the spiritual development process.

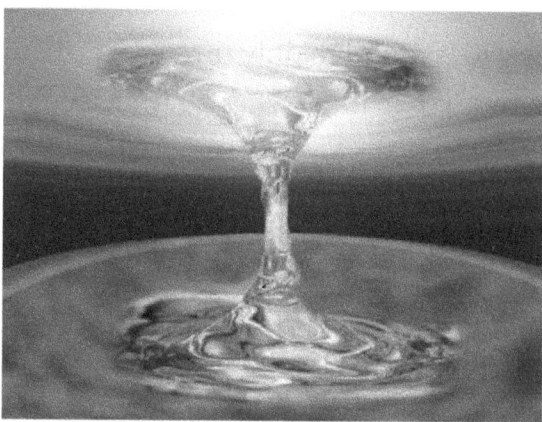

The Importance of Stillness

How does spiritual growth help one stay healthy; and what is stillness?

The ideas I'm going to discuss here relate to eastern Asian concepts of the spirit as taught mainly in China and India.

Buddhism, Taoism, Zen, and other eastern religions and philosophies all teach that the spirit is the core of our being; and that our physical bodies are just an extension of that spirit into the physical level of existence.

By learning to let your mind or ego release its hold on the illusion of our current existence, we become aware of the spirit behind or at the core of our being. This spirit is the pure oneness of God and exists in no time and no space. (A concept which we really can't envision with our minds or egos only).

There are many techniques taught to get closer to realizing the core of a person's being. These techniques all involve practicing spiritual growth, love, and/or meditation with a goal of enlightenment.

There are thousands of books and practices on this subject so I will not try to duplicate them in this short synopsis.

The Chinese stress that the stillness and oneness obtained through spiritual growth are one of the main keys to keeping the body healthy for a long life. Many Taoist techniques and teachings stress the achievement of "stillness" as a prelude to physical immortality.

The stillness I'm referring to is found mainly through meditation. In Christian terms it is often referred to as the "Peace that passes all understanding".

It is hard to describe the feeling of stillness since it is like when you first wake up in the morning after a deep sleep—but even quieter and deeper.

The feeling of stillness has a strong effect on your body—it seems to make the randomness of your cells quiet down into a more restful state.

Meditation is taught many places; I've even found a company called Holosync (24) which sells CDs that help even beginners achieve deep states of relaxation that usually takes advanced Yogis years of practice

Stillness is not something achieved overnight but takes years, (even with modern advanced CD techniques) to start showing results.

However, the effects of stillness practices probably have the most profound effects on your body's aging as anything else recommended in this book.

This is since as you start to achieve stillness, your Ego is realizing its core is really part of the spirit— not a separate mind. The spirit exists outside time and space. This connection with your spirit has a profound health effect on the body in terms of peace and wellbeing.

When meditating in this state you can feel stillness penetrating your body.

It feels like your body is reaching a relaxed state never realized; even in sleep.

The state of the stillness of your spirit provides a modified blueprint for your body's health.

It is a lot of work to set aside time every day to meditate. The good news is you will find that after some weeks of practicing, this time becomes something you look forward to. This is since meditation is so relaxing it becomes a way to recharge you for daily activities in the world.

I also find that meditation makes my mind more alert when I wake up in the morning and gives me a sharper intellectual edge at work.

Your Spiritual, Energy, and Physical Bodies

One of the key concepts in this book is that you are not just your physical body.

These are concepts which are woven into many religions and philosophies, with related energy body concepts mostly being understood in the East more than the West.

Many believe that your entire being consists of at least three states as described below. The Spirit

Here we mean the spirit which is your "soul" or core of your being. An individual's spirit is one with the God spirit and is present in every person and every being. It exists outside of time and space. This is a place some call "no time and no space". It is everywhere present simultaneously.

The spirit exists in all things and each person has that same core spirit within them.

We can learn to live focused more in the spirit through a variety of religious, meditational, and philosophical traditions.

A Direct Connection between stillness practices and the long term health of our bodies.

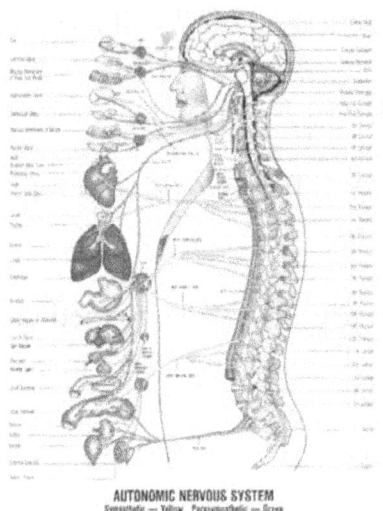
AUTONOMIC NERVOUS SYSTEM
Sympathetic — Yellow Parasympathetic — Green

The Anterior Nervous System can be controlled and our bodies health stabilized for the Long Term through spiritual practices

Aging is a health continuum. It is a delicate balance between nutrition and healing versus body deterioration. As the body ages, the function of the cells in the body decline at various rates. As cell function declines, cells become vulnerable to stress.

Cell "stress" includes processed and fatty foods, environmental toxins, poor sleep, negative life stress (both physical and emotional), and excessive weight gain. Stressors illicit slow and chronic inflammation. There are different types of inflammation. There is a healthy acute inflammatory reaction in response to injury which starts and maintains the repair process. There is another type of inflammation which is chronic and slow. This is a different type of response which causes damage to the body.

Chronic inflammation plays a role in premature cell death and the development of chronic disease. Chronic Disease is defined as a long-lasting condition that can be controlled but not cured. Chronic illnesses include diabetes, obesity, heart disease, cancer, arthritis and other autoimmune diseases.

According to the Center for Disease Control, chronic disease is the leading cause of death and disability in the United States and 75% of US health care $ goes to the treatment of these diseases.

The number of individuals with one or more chronic diseases, as well as the cost for treatment of these conditions, is estimated to dramatically increase during the next 5 years.

Some sources state that the body is in a constant inflammatory state and that the individual can decrease the rate of cell aging thru lifestyle. Nutrition and physical activity are both very important. Our genes also play a role. The organs in the body are controlled by the autonomic nervous system (ANS).

The ANS controls involuntary actions (such as heart beat, digestion) and is made of the nerves that relax the body [Parasympathetic Nervous System (PNS)] and nerves that respond to stress [Sympathetic Nervous System (SNS)]. There is a balance between the PNS and SNS. For the body to be in a good autonomic nervous state, the PNS should be more active than the SNS. The control station of the ANS is the brain.

The stressors that promote inflammation, also negatively affect the ANS. This imbalance can be improved by nutrition, physical activity and spiritual practices, such as meditation and prayer.

An example of the potential powerful effect of meditation has been demonstrated by a male client of the group. He is in his late 50's, has Diabetes Type 2, arthritis of a hip and is obese. He meditates daily and has been working with meditation for many years. Despite the negative stressors his body is confronted with, his ANS was in perfect balance.

As the ANS affects every organ in the body this is a great basis for any life style improvement. Here is a link to an article with more details on this subject:

<u>Use of Complementary and Alternative Medicine Among Patients With Arthritis</u>

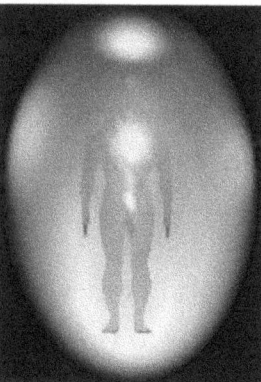

The Energy Body

Some organizations like the Hindus and Theosophists believe we have multiple energy body levels. The Theosophists believe there are at least six distinct energy bodies.

Many other traditions only talk about one energy body which provides the life force to energize our physical bodies.

The acupuncture meridians and chakras are all parts of the energy body which exists in very close proximity to the physical body.

The aura is also a manifestation of the energy body too, which overlaps your physical body.

Many people claim to be able to see "auras" including this Author. The aura is the physical energy manifestation of the energy body. All living people have an aura and one can tell a lot about their health by how their aura looks.

The Physical Body

This is the body most of us know, and that most of us think is all of us that exists. This is the body we want to heal and energize to achieve physical immortality.

Exercises done on the physical body also affect the energy body.

Herbal supplements work from the physical body to help correct energy flows in your energy body. How the Bodies Work Together

The concept of the spiritual development exercises, and physical exercises in this book is that they help increase the synchronization of these bodies.

By bringing the absolute peace and stillness of the spirit down into the energy and physical bodies you increase the perfection and health of those bodies.

This is since in the normal course of events the stresses of our life cause more randomness or entropy in our energy and physical bodies. These stresses of daily life age us prematurely and cause disease.

We can repair our energy and physical bodies by integrating them better with the spiritual body; and getting the energies to flow in the correct patterns, chakras, and meridians, and with more vital force.

A Course in Miracles

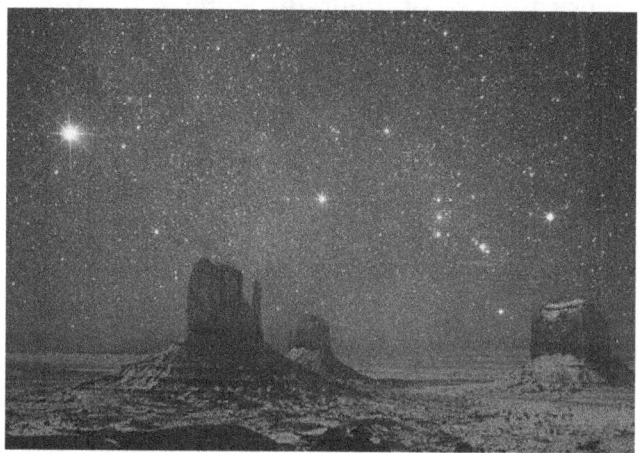

I would be remiss to end this section on our spiritual connection without mentioning "A Course in Miracles" which has been published and disseminated since 1975 by the Foundation for Inner Peace.

The best explanation of the course comes from their website:

> *This is a course in miracles. It is a required course. Only the time you take it is voluntary. Free will does not mean that you can establish the curriculum. It means only that you can elect what you want to take at a given time. The course does not aim at teaching the meaning of love, for that is beyond what can be taught. It does aim, however, at removing the blocks to the awareness of love's presence, which is your natural inheritance. The opposite of love is fear, but what is all-encompassing can have no opposite.*

This course can therefore be summed up very simply in this way:

> *Nothing real can be threatened. Nothing unreal exists.*
> *Herein lies the peace of God.*

I did the course for about six months and found it was an excellent tool to help me become more centered and develop more stillness.

I had often felt in recent years that old thoughts, fears, and stresses were building up in my mind like dirt or crud, and were causing my spirit to be covered by a fog or cotton candy which made me less clear and not able to think as well.

One day I remember I was working on the Course in Miracles lessons and suddenly it felt like a large part of this shell of mentally accreted garbage suddenly came apart and sloughed off my spirit. It was a physical experience.

An analogy might be a heavy coat of dirt and grime coming off a car after a good wash so that the bright colors and shininess of the car comes through again.

This course is another tool for spiritual growth which can help you get better connected to your spiritual core as part of the physical immortality process.

Chapter Summary

In this chapter we covered some explanations of the reality of the eternal spirit, and how stillness practices help our body.

The synchronization of our spiritual, vital forces, and physical bodies is important to our long term health.

I've also met many other holistic practitioners who have come to the same conclusions as me about our three bodies, and they believe as I do about addressing all three for long term health.

Another area of the spiritual experience is what we call "unconditional love".

It is so important to our health and happiness that I thought it should be it's own principle of personal longevity.

6.0 Having Love In Your Heart

Everything that exists is both hunter and prey.
What is it that we hunt? Humans hunt for love.
We feel that we need that love, because we believe we don't have love,
because we don't love ourselves.
We hunt for love in other humans just like us,
expecting to get love from them when these
humans are in the condition as we are.
We are hunting for love, when the love we need is inside ourselves.
-Don Miguel Ruiz

The fifth principle of personal longevity is Unconditional Love.

Unconditional Love (UL) is something I only really experienced in the last couple of years.

UL is of course related to our general spiritual connection, but its essence is something very powerful which improves our overall happiness, immune system, and connection with others.

This chapter discusses all the types of love, and then focuses on understanding unconditional love and how to experience it in your life.

Let's start with some definitions of different types of love:

What is Love?

We all know something about love because the reality permeates our daily lives. But something is missing in our daily lives—and we don't know why.

We may feel that we don't have enough love:

- That we are not loved
- That we are not worthy of being loved
- That someone who loved us no longer feels the same

- That love within our own families may not be the same that it used to be
- That other people are loved more than us.

Or we may feel very happy sometimes:

- The happiness of being with our significant other—girlfriend, boyfriend, or spouse
- The love we have as parents for children
- The love for pets
- The spiritual love for total strangers
- The love for a city, state, country, or humanity in general

In any event, the feelings of love go silent—why can't we always be happy with love?

To get a better handle on how love affects our lives, we should also understand the different types of love we experience.

C.S.Lewis wrote one of the definitive classics on love titled "The Four Loves"; covering the subject of Love and he defined that four types of Love exist.

The types of Love C.S. Lewis defines in Greek with their English words are:

Storge-Affection

What people feel for family members and others they may have themselves together by chance. It is the most natural and widely diffused of the loves.

Philia-Friendship

This is love between friends. Friendship is a strong bond existing between persons who share common interests or activities. It's the least biological, organic, instinctive, and necessary of the four Loves.

Eros-Romance

Eros is about being in Love or loving another. This is separate from sexuality although the two are often related.

Agape-Unconditional Love

Agape is the most unconditional love which can happen no matter what the circumstance. It is often stressed as a Christian virtue although agape is not specific to any religion and can be experienced by anyone.

****

Love and Affection

Love begins from birth and can be easily carried out throughout life by the human necessity of affection. People strive and live for lasting affection. It is healthy to feel emotions and feel nurtured. Through these states of feeling, love can be brought forward in a positive manner. So positive in fact that affectionate behavior is linked to many health benefits.

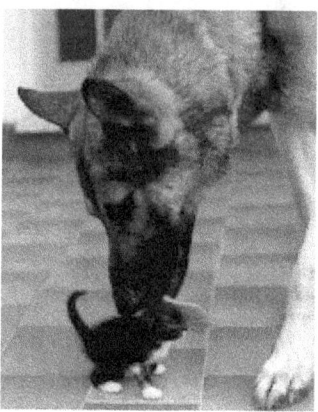

According to psychologist Henry Murray, there are five types of affection needs. These include affiliation, nurturance, play, rejection, and succorance.

Examples of these types of affections include the following:

- Spending time with other people
- Taking care of another person
- Having fun with others
- Rejecting other people
- Being helped or protected by others

These affection needs are both on a conscious and unconscious level, just as our love for others can be. Ask yourself if you are participating in the 5 types of affection. What areas may you be lacking in?

Acknowledge your truth for you have just discovered what may or may not be missing links to your own pleasantness, pleasure, and displeasure. Once having realized this, you are then able to take charge with how you want to feel with yourself, especially in direct relation to love.

Are you experiencing tension or relaxation? Excitement or depression?

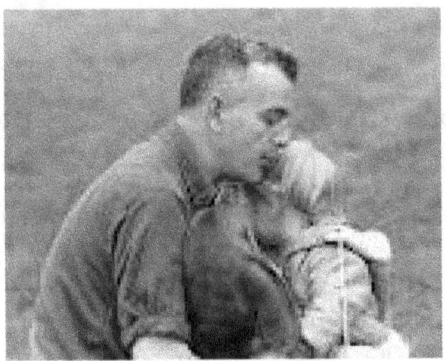

Having answered these questions and digesting your answers, dig deep into the 5 types of affection and fill in those blocks one step at a time. Keep track of the small steps you make toward becoming a well-rounded, affectionate person. Thank yourself and others. Feel gratitude around you. You have the power to feel and express your love. You are love!

Feeling the love today?? Reach out to someone special or perhaps someone you have been wanting to connect with lately. JM

Love and Friendship

Without friends, love is nonexistent. Love is eternal and unconditional through the relationship with a strong friend. Friendship can be eternal through knowing someone on such a deep level that forms through trust, listening to one another, and experiencing new ways of life. It is important to find compatibility when choosing our best friends, wisely, through the psychological and emotional levels we know as ourselves.

After all, a friendship can many times be summed up to what Aristotle quotes, "What is a friend? A single soul, dwelling in two bodies." A true friend can be formed through one warm heart reaching out to another. Love is found through those feelings of empathy and sympathy that forms the bond between lasting friendships.

6.0 Having Love In Your Heart

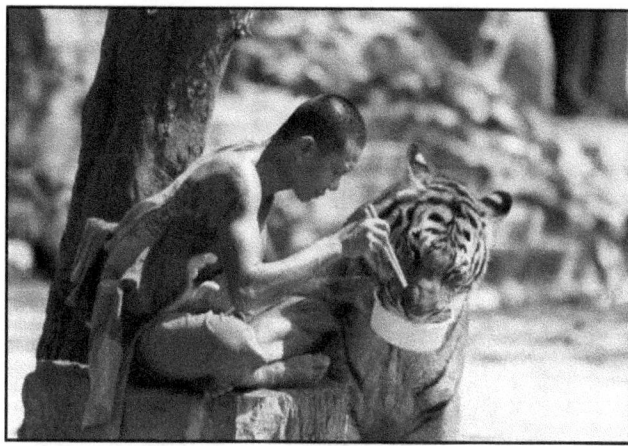

So how can love be formed through friendship? Below is a list of popular answers taken from well known books and quotes from people:

Friendship is a sweet attraction of the heart, towards the merit we esteem, or the "perfections we admire; and produces a mutual inclination between two persons, to promote each other's interest, knowledge, virtue, and happiness."- Wellins Calott

"Some people come into our lives and quickly go. Some stay for a while and leave footprints on our hearts. And we are never, ever the same." –Unknown

"Friendship involves many things, but above all, the power of going out of one's self and appreciating what is noble and loving in another." –Thomas Hughes

"There is a magnet in your heart that will attract true friends. That magnet is unselfishness, thinking of others first…when you learn to live for others, they will live for you." –Paramahansa Yogananda

"No love, no friendship can cross the path of our destiny without leaving some mark on it forever." – Francois Mauriac

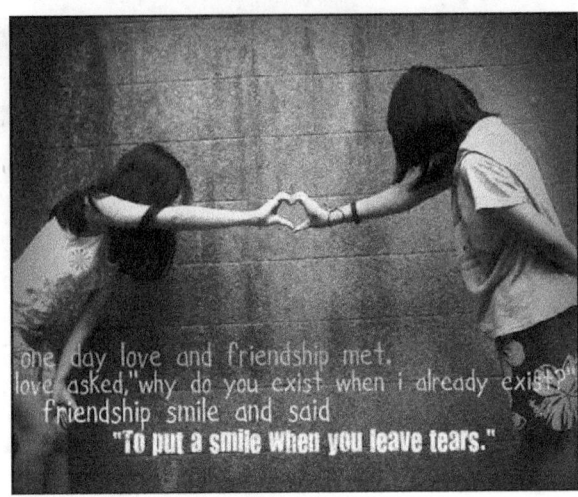

I hope these quotes leave you with a warm heart and you are able to move forward in your friendships with others, and most importantly, your friendship to yourself!

JM

Love and Romance

We have all experienced love in many forms with different people, animals, and even hobbies. But what about romantic love? Romance is defined by Webster as "A love affair."

An emotional involvement takes place between two people and their time can be shared with one another in enthusiasm, mystery, pleasure and fascination. If these feelings are formed and bonded between the two, a spiritual relationship may also unfold into a romantic relationship filled with even more love and meaning.

6.0 Having Love In Your Heart

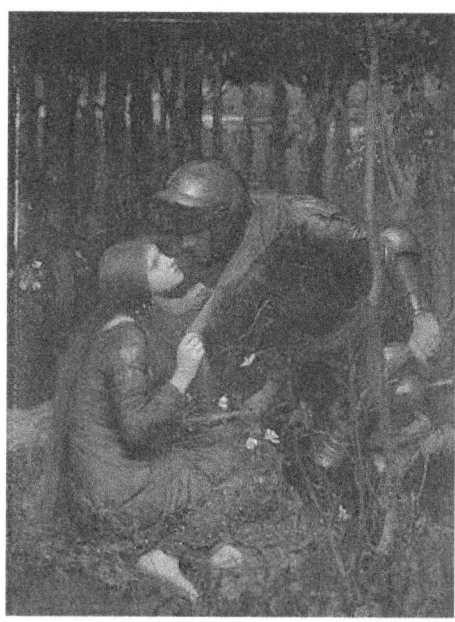

"People compose poetry, novels, sitcoms for love," says Helen Fisher, anthropologist at Rutgers University. "They live for love, die for love, kill for love. It can be stronger than the drive to stay alive."

Listed below are some of the key factors for a successful romantic relationship:

- Tell your partner you love them
- Be there for your partner
- Show affection and share yourself
- Give gifts to show you care
- Allow "alone time" for yourself
- Take no-thing for granted

What are some of the things you have done for others that affected them in a positive way? Think about your strength as a person and how you can utilize your gifts to others.'

"You don't love someone for their looks, or their clothes, or for their fancy car, but because they sing a song only you can hear."

To the beauty of romance, JM

Love Defined Through Quotes

Sometimes one of the best ways to understand Love is to contemplate quotes by famous people on the subject. Here are some of our favorites to meditate on…

10 Quotes on Love

Here are some wonderful words put together from a few brilliant minds. Along with the quotes are some pictures to feel the soul. Enjoy <3

(NAD does not claim rights to any of the pictures posted.)

"Love is the beauty of the soul." St. Aurelius Augustine

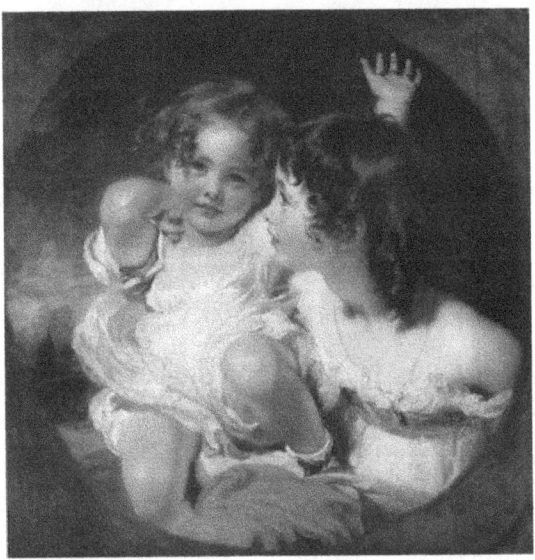

"If the sight of the blue skies fills you with joy, if a blade of grass springing up in the fields has power to move you, if the simple things of nature have a message that you understand, rejoice, for your soul is alive…"Eleonora Duse

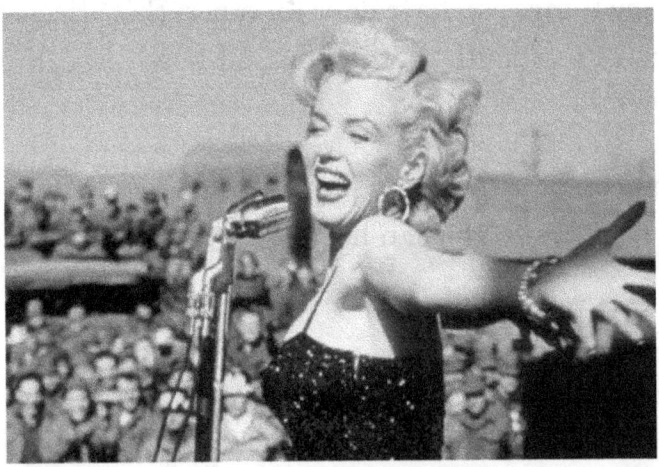

"Harmony is pure love, for love is a concerto." Lope de Vega

"The best and most beautiful things in the world cannot be seen or even touched. They must be felt with the heart." Helen Keller

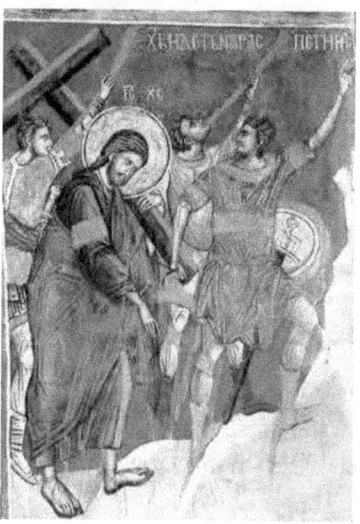

"There is only one happiness in life, to love and be loved." George Sand

"And, when he shall die, take him and cut him out in little stars, and he will make the face of Heaven so fine that all the world will be in love with night and pay no worship to the garish sun." {Romeo and Juliet} – William Shakespeare

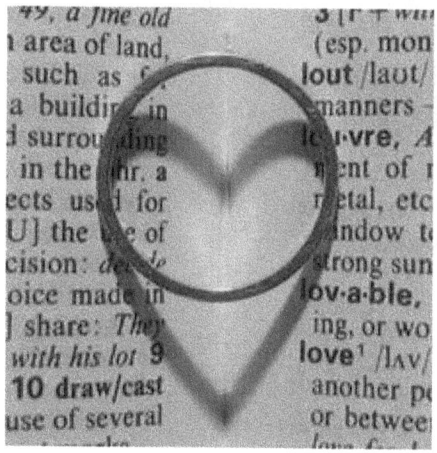

"You come to love not by finding the perfect person, but by learning to see an imperfect person perfectly." Sam Keen

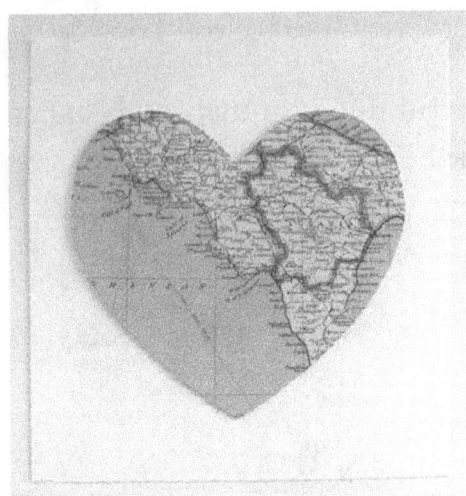

"Too often we underestimate the power of a touch, a smile, a kind word, a listening ear, an honest compliment, or the smallest act of caring, all of which have the potential to turn a life around." Leo Buscaglia

"True love stories never have endings. "Richard Bach

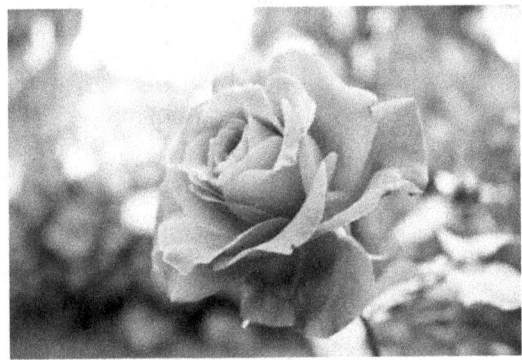

"The heart is the only constant and sure beam to follow ones cosmic door of understanding." Mentor, Agartha

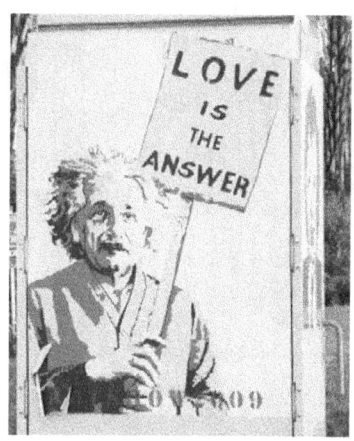

JM

Unconditional Love:

Unconditional Love is a very spiritual state and most of us experience it rarely in our lives-if at all.

If you can improve the force of love acting in your life and get an uplifted attitude from reading this material—then I will have accomplished my goal.

Love in the Bible (Various, The Holy Bible)

The Holy Bible is the core teaching of Christianity and stresses Love for spiritual growth and happiness in one's life.

Jesus taught about loving God in many different ways and the Old and New Testaments provide many of the most famous quotes on love.

Several quotes illustrate the themes of love in the Bible including unconditional love which we will focus on later in this book.

Probably the most famous quote on love in the Bible is used today in many weddings and refers to what we call unconditional love:

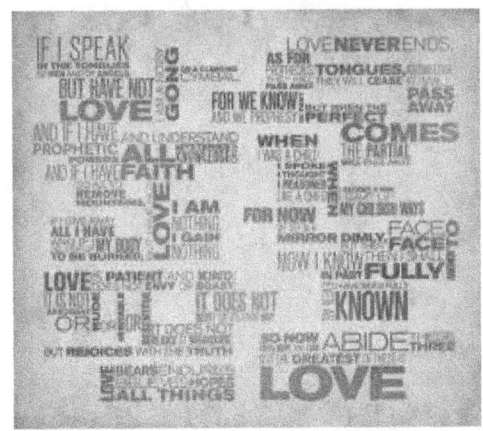

1 Corinthians 13:4-13 *Love is patient and kind; love does not envy or boast; it is not arrogant or rude. It does not insist on its own way; it is not irritable or resentful-it does not rejoice at wrongdoing, but rejoices with the truth. Love bears all things, believes all things, hopes all things, endures all things. Love never ends.* As for prophecies, they will pass away; as for tongues, they will cease; as for knowledge, it will pass away. For we know in part and we prophesy in part, but when the perfect comes, the partial will pass away. When I was a child, I spoke like a child, I thought like a child, I reasoned like a child. When I became a man, I gave up childish ways. For now we see in a mirror dimly, but then face to face. Now I know in part; then I shall know fully, even as I have been fully known. So now faith, hope, and love abide, these three; but the greatest of these is love.

Another quote on loving your enemies implies a spiritual and unattached love which is above the "normal" types of love:

Luke 6:35
But love your enemies, do good to them, and lend to them without expecting to get anything back. Then your reward will be great, and you will be sons of the Most High, because he is kind to the ungrateful and wicked.

Love has the benefit of overcoming fear:

> 1 John 4:18-19
> There is no fear in love. But perfect love drives out fear, because fear has to do with punishment. The one who fears is not made perfect in love. We love because he first loved us.

Another way of visualizing unconditional love:

> Song of Solomon 8:4-8 Daughters of Jerusalem, I charge you: Do not arouse or awaken love until it so desires. Who is this coming up from the desert leaning on her lover? Under the apple tree I roused you; there your mother conceived you, there she who was in labor gave you birth. *Place me like a seal over your heart, like a seal on your arm; for love is as strong as death, its jealousy unyielding as the grave. It burns like blazing fire, like a mighty flame. Many waters cannot quench love; rivers cannot wash it away. If one were to give all the wealth of his house for love*, it would be utterly scorned. We have a young sister, and her breasts are not yet grown. What shall we do for our sister for the day she is spoken for?

How else can we love all our neighbors except with the love of God?

> Matthew 22:37-39
> Jesus replied: "Love the Lord your God with all your heart and with all your soul and with all your mind." This is the first and greatest commandment. And the second is like it: 'Love your neighbor as yourself.'

More on Unconditional LOVE

Part of Unconditional Love is learning to love yourself—not in an egoic sense, but in terms of loving who you are, your qualities, your good points and your faults—total acceptance of who you are.

Unconditional LOVE... Surrounding you and your being... Surrounding Every-Thing around you. This love is including physically, spiritually, emotionally, and mentally.

THIS IS YOUR LIFE.
DO WHAT YOU LOVE, AND DO IT OFTEN.
IF YOU DON'T LIKE SOMETHING, CHANGE IT.
IF YOU DON'T LIKE YOUR JOB, QUIT.
IF YOU DON'T HAVE ENOUGH TIME, STOP WATCHING TV.
IF YOU ARE LOOKING FOR THE LOVE OF YOUR LIFE, STOP;
THEY WILL BE WAITING FOR YOU WHEN YOU
START DOING THINGS YOU LOVE.
STOP OVER ANALYZING, ALL EMOTIONS ARE BEAUTIFUL.
LIFE IS SIMPLE. WHEN YOU EAT, APPRECIATE EVERY LAST BITE.
OPEN YOUR MIND, ARMS, AND HEART TO NEW THINGS AND PEOPLE, WE ARE UNITED IN OUR DIFFERENCES.
ASK THE NEXT PERSON YOU SEE WHAT THEIR PASSION IS, AND SHARE YOUR INSPIRING DREAM WITH THEM.
TRAVEL OFTEN; GETTING LOST WILL HELP YOU FIND YOURSELF.
SOME OPPORTUNITIES ONLY COME ONCE, SEIZE THEM.
LIFE IS ABOUT THE PEOPLE YOU MEET, AND THE THINGS YOU CREATE WITH THEM
SO GO OUT AND START CREATING.
LIFE IS SHORT. LIVE YOUR DREAM, AND WEAR YOUR PASSION.

"The only way love can last a lifetime is if it's unconditional. The truth is this: love is not determined by the one being loved but rather by the one choosing to love."

This beautiful quote is by Stephen Kendrick and is has an underlying truth to it; we are the ones who get to choose our love. We choose our destiny. Everything around us is our choice and we are capable of being as loving as we want to be!

Spreading the love is important and reflects who we are on the inside and outside. If we are able to have a fine outlook on our life, future, and goals, being able to move forward with each step in grace and positivity, our inward selves are being loved. If you are at a good place in your life, keep it going! Spread it forward. Let the love you shine last a lifetime.

What loving things are you grateful for? Making a daily list of 5 things you are grateful for and reflecting back on it in moments of solitude, meditation, or even when you are down, can be a great form of healing the self.

Today, my list contains the following five:

- I am grateful to have fingers to type and express Unconditional LOVE.
- I am grateful I have food to eat tonight.
- I am grateful for my job.
- I am grateful to be at peace with my inner being.
- I am grateful to have talked to my dad on the phone today.

What are your five?? Make a list and share with us.. Let's spread the love forward. "When the power of love is greater than the love of power, the world will know peace" Love, love, love, JM

The Story of Ram Dass

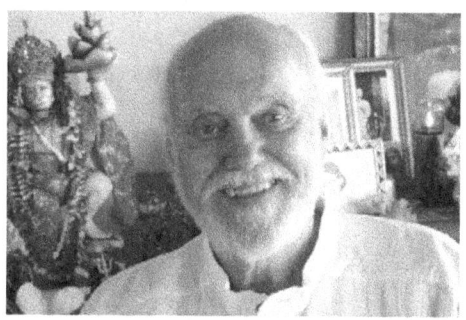

Ram Dass was born as Richard Alpert on April 6, 1931. He is an American contemporary spiritual teacher and the author of the very famous 1971 book *"Be Here Now"*.

I found a lot of quotes from this book on Unconditional Love which are very helpful to a better understanding that state and how to achieve it.

Ram Dass is also known for his personal and professional associations with Timothy Leary at Harvard University in the early 1960s, for his travels to India and his relationship with the Hindu guru Neem Karoli Baba, and for founding the charitable organizations Seva Foundation and Hanuman Foundation.

Ram Dass also wrote several other books including one called:

"Be Love Now-The Path of the Heart"

Ram Dass had many things to tell the world about the opening of his heart. His personal experience in how he first started to feel unconditional love from his master is insightful:

Years ago in India I was sitting in the courtyard of the little temple in the Himalayan foothills. Thirty or forty of us were there around my guru, Maharaj-ji. This old man wrapped in a plaid blanket was sitting on a plank bed, and for a brief uncommon interval everyone had fallen silent. It was a meditative quiet, like an open field on a windless day or a deep clear lake without a ripple. I felt waves of love radiating toward me, washing over me like a gentle surf on a tropical shore, immersing me, rocking me, caressing my soul, infinitely accepting and open. I was nearly overcome, on the verge of tears, so grateful and so full of joy it was hard to believe it was happening. I opened my eyes and looked around, and I could feel that everyone else around me was experiencing the same thing. I looked over at my guru. He was just sitting there, looking around, not doing anything. It was just his being, shining like the sun equally on everyone. It wasn't directed at anyone in particular. For him it was nothing special, just his own nature.

Ram Dass went on to become a famous teacher of enlightenment himself and a devotee of the ways of living in the now of love.

Paths to Unconditional Love

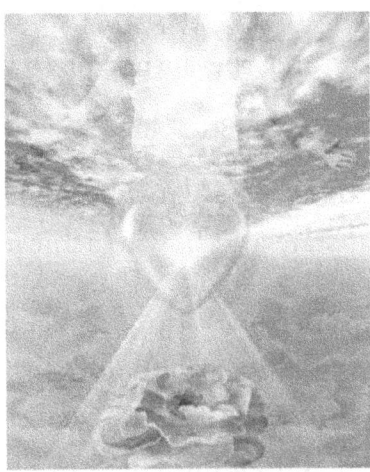

Now let's look at how unconditional love is described and the ways it can be achieved.

My first experience with feeling a strong presence of unconditional love was the result of practicing the heart rose meditation. (shown later in this chapter)

As a result of this exercise my heart chakra opened and I felt this intense love force emanating from me to everyone and everything around me. It was like to most intense feelings of being in love with someone but it was directed outward to everything in my surroundings.

Feelings like this are hard to describe since they are a type of spiritual ecstasy.

The first experience lasted a few hours—a real natural high. Have had that experience a few times since, and learning to feel like that every waking moment is my goal.

Ram Dass recounts his first experience with unconditional love here:

The first time you experience unconditional love as an adult, it may be a gentle melting of a glacier. Or it may be more of a cataclysm, like a giant earthquake that shakes you to your inner core. You are falling in love, but the act of receiving love that intense and all-encompassing changes your conception of yourself. You can't swim in such a vast ocean and remain entirely in the small pond of your limited self. Even if that opening is only for an instant, even if it goes away and is apparently forgotten, that moment of realization, of the heart opening, colors the rest of a lifetime. There's no going back. The lingering taste of that ultimate sweetness remains and won't be denied.

Dass, Ram; Das, Rameshwar. Be Love Now: The Path of the Heart (p. 4). Harper Collins, Inc... Kindle Edition.

What is this state of love then?

Love is actually a state of being, and a divine state at that, the state to which we all yearn to return. The outer love object stimulates a feeling of love, but the love is inside us. We interpret it as coming

from outside us, so we want to possess love, and we reach outside for something that is already inside us.

Dass, Ram; Das, Rameshwar (2010-11-02). Be Love Now: The Path of the Heart (p. 15). Harper Collins, Inc.. Kindle Edition.

And how does this affect your ego?

You don't kill your ego; you kill your identification with your ego. As you dissolve into love, your ego fades. You're not thinking about loving; you're just being love, radiating like the sun. That last step requires Grace.

Dass, Ram; Das, Rameshwar (2010-11-02). Be Love Now: The Path of the Heart (p. 27). Harper Collins, Inc.. Kindle Edition.

What is surrender in this context?

In the West surrender implies giving up power. But surrendering to a guru or the Beloved doesn't mean giving power to another human being— it's letting go of the stuff that keeps you separate. Each time you surrender, it leads you further in, deeper into yourself. You surrender to that place in yourself that takes you beyond form.

Dass, Ram; Das, Rameshwar (2010-11-02). Be Love Now: The Path of the Heart (pp. 57-58). Harper Collins, Inc.. Kindle Edition.

What is the goal of this love?

Although you may devote yourself to an aspect of the Beloved, like the guru or the deity as mother, child, or lover, you are in it for the love, not for the attainment, not for the object. It's one of those wonderful paradoxes you encounter on the path. You can't attain it; you have to become it. In the process subject and object, lover and Beloved, become one. You lose yourself and gain your Self. To go from the experiencer to the merger with the One requires grace. Know that when you learn to lose yourself, you will reach the beloved. There is no other secret to be learned, and more than this is not known to me. —Ansari of Herat10

Dass, Ram; Das, Rameshwar (2010-11-02). Be Love Now: The Path of the Heart (p. 61). Harper Collins, Inc.. Kindle Edition.

Although you may devote yourself to an aspect of the Beloved, like the guru or the deity as mother, child, or lover, you are in it for the love, not for the attainment, not for the object. It's one of those wonderful paradoxes you encounter on the path. You can't attain it; you

Dass, Ram; Das, Rameshwar (2010-11-02). Be Love Now: The Path of the Heart (p. 61). Harper Collins, Inc.. Kindle Edition.

7.0 Exercises in Unconditional Love

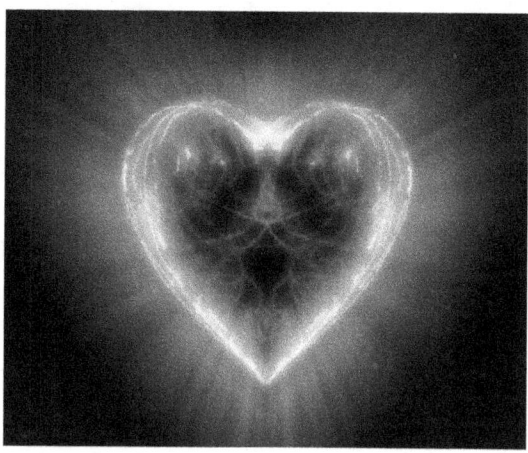

A Loving Kindness Meditation:

This first exercise is a basic meditational exercise designed to improve your happiness and attitude throughout the day and help get you ready for deeper exercises on experiencing unconditional love:

Sit on the ground in a comfortable position (lotus position isn't necessary, but is optimal) with your back straight. I've found that sitting on two pillows makes meditation MUCH more comfortable, so try that out if you're finding it too painful.

Close your eyes. Relax your entire body. Let go of any unnecessary tension in your muscles, and stop thinking about whatever it is you're thinking about. Allow your mind to drift to wherever it likes for *a minute* or so.

Next, focus completely on the inhalation and exhalation of your breath for *1 minute*. This isn't a breath control exercise, so don't attempt to change your breath in any way. Just observe the natural inflow and outflow of your breath *as it is*.

Now, recite in your mind **"May *I* be happy. May *I* be peaceful. May *I* be free from misery, animosity, judgment, and negativity."**• Pause between each statement, and *feel* the power of what you've just recited. Absorb yourself in feelings of happiness, peace, and Love. I like to imagine an immense amount of Love energy flowing into my body from my external environment while doing this step of the exercise.

Next, recite in your mind, **"May all beings be happy. May all beings be peaceful. May all beings be free from misery, animosity, judgment, and negativity."**• Once again, pause between each statement and *feel* the power of what you've just recited. When I do this, I imagine the faces of as many people as I possibly can, and I send each person a powerful intention of Love. I send this intention by imagining my Love as a tremendous wave of energy flowing out of my abdominal area. Repeat this process 3-4 times.

Next, recite in your mind, **"May all beings share in my merits, good deeds, compassion, kindness, positive energy, patience, generosity, and Love."**• Keep emitting powerful waves of Love energy while reciting this statement in your mind.

Finally, recite in your mind, **"May all beings I have hurt in the past forgive me for doing so. May *I* also forgive all beings who have hurt me in the past."**• This is my favorite step of the exercise, because I almost always experience an immediate and substantial release of negative energy. I try to pull up the images of the people that I have hurt and who have hurt me, and I imagine us hugging and getting along with one another. I feel the Loving connection we now share between us.

Open your eyes. You're done!

A Shift Into the Heart

The below passage and exercise is from the book "Living from the Heart" which helps one focus consciousness in the heart as a first step towards getting to the experience of unconditional love…

THE SHIFT INTO THE HEART The center of your chest, which is next to your physical heart, is often considered the spiritual center of your Being. For many centuries, it was believed that thinking happened in the heart rather than in the brain. What would it be like to experience the world from this energetic center instead of from the head? What effect would that have on your experience of the world and of yourself?

Exercise: Try this exercise first with your eyes closed and then open. Notice what you are aware of in this moment: the sounds, a thought, the objects around you. Notice if you are looking or listening or sensing from the head, and notice what that is like. Now gently drop your sensing down into your Heart.

This is not a matter of sensing the Heart or feeling what is in your Heart, but feeling your surroundings from the center of your chest. At first, it can be helpful to rest your hand on the center of your chest next to your heart, to help orient yourself to looking from this place. Allow what you are seeing to be seen by your Heart instead of your head. What is it like to sense, listen, and look from your Heart?

Pick an object and sense it with your Heart instead of your head. How is that?

Nirmala (2009-02-15). Living from the Heart (Kindle Locations 416-420). Endless Satsang Foundation. Kindle Edition.

Heart Rose Meditation:

I've had great results from this exercise and it resulted in my first strong feelings of unconditional love—which lasted for hours…

The objectives of this exercise are to:

To find your spiritual heart center

To start the gradual process of opening your spiritual heart center

Kindly imagine a flower inside your heart. Suppose you refer a rose. Imagine that the rose is not fully blossomed; it is still a bud. After you meditated for two or three minutes, please try to imagine that petal by petal the flower is blossoming.

See and feel the flower blossoming petal by petal inside your heart. Then, after 5 minutes, try to feel that there is no heart all; there is only a flower inside your heart. You do not have a heart, but only a flower. The flower has become your heart or your heart has become a flower.

After 7 or 8 minutes, please feel that this flower-heart has covered your whole body. Your body is no longer here; from your head to your feet you can feel the fragrance of the rose. If you look at your feet, immediately you experience the fragrance of the rose. If you look at your knee, you experience the fragrance of the rose. If you look at your hand, you experience the fragrance of the rose.

Everywhere there is beauty, fragrance and purity of the rose have permeated your entire body.

Just as you can concentrate on the tip of your finger, or a candle or any other material object, you can also concentrate on your heart. You may close your eyes or look at a wall, but all the time you are thinking of your heart as a dear friend. When this thinking becomes most intense, when it absorbs your entire attention, then you have gone beyond ordinary thinking and entered into concentration. You cannot look physically at your spiritual heart, but you can focus all your attention on it. Then gradually the power of your concentration enters into the heart and takes completely out of the realm of the mind.

To reach your spiritual heart you have to feel you don't have a mind, you do not have arms, you do not have legs, you only have a heart. Then you have to feel you do not have the heart, but that you are the heart. When you can feel that you are the heart and nothing else, then easily you will be able to reach your spiritual heart during your meditation.

Key points of the Exercise:

*Visualize the flower clearly at the beginning

*Bring the Flower into your heart Center, Identify with it so you do not feel any separation from it.

Loving in the Now

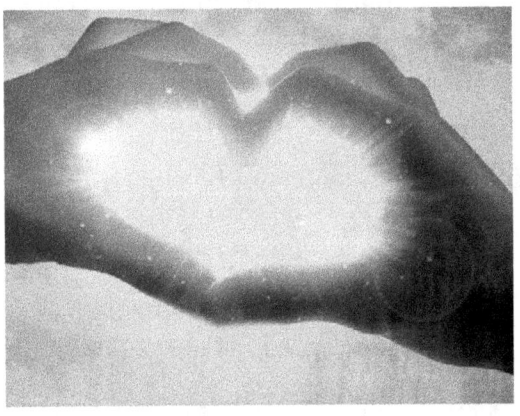

So what do we mean by "Loving in the Now"? (Nirmala)

This is all about the shift in consciousness required to experience unconditional love. The normal path is to first quiet the mind through meditational and relaxation practices.

Once this cultivated peace of mind becomes a normal part of your life, then you can work on opening your heart chakra through exercises like the Hear Rose Meditation.

It is the opening of the heart and the re-focusing of your presence and consciousness into the heart which helps one to start experiencing the presence of God.

God is the universal energy or force of love, so once we can attune ourselves to that presence we start to feel oneness with God—which is the universal source of unconditional love.

Why is this such a great spiritual state to reach? Because when we do, we live in joy, and the thoughts which might draw us into a "downer" state no longer affect us.

Living in this state all of the time lets us process the daily events of our life through a positive and loving prism.

We think about joy in our lives—not about pain and unhappiness.

This is the goal of enlightenment—to live in the world with all of its attachments and pain—but not let the core of your being be affected.

To live in an unending state of joy which helps all of our relationships and friendships to have a more joyous and positive outcome.

"Living From the Heart" also has some great points about awareness from the heart while living in the now:

IT IS ALL DIVINE NATURE The experience of looking from the Heart is quite different from looking from the head, but the looking itself is fundamentally the same. To contact your Being, it isn't necessary to look from the Heart or from anywhere in particular. While it's much easier to contact the nature of your Being when you look from the Heart, even when it is flowing less fully, it is still your true nature.

The point of these exercises is to show you the nature of your Being so thoroughly that you can rest as that aware space. Experiencing more fully the limitless nature of your Being is freeing. Discovering that this is always the nature of your Being, no matter what is shaping or limiting your experience of it, is even more freeing. You can rest in this essential awareness no matter what is happening or how you are experiencing it. Just as you don't need to see your car to know it exists, you don't need to have a rich and full experience of your Being in every moment to know it exists. It is always here. It's what is living you.

This alive awareness and spaciousness is the nature of you. It is your divine nature. You are divine. Even when you are contracted and confused, you are divine. It's all divine. That is all there is, and you are that.

Nirmala (2009-02-15). Living from the Heart (pp. 81-82). Endless Satsang Foundation. Kindle Edition.

Imagine the Greatest Love in Your Life

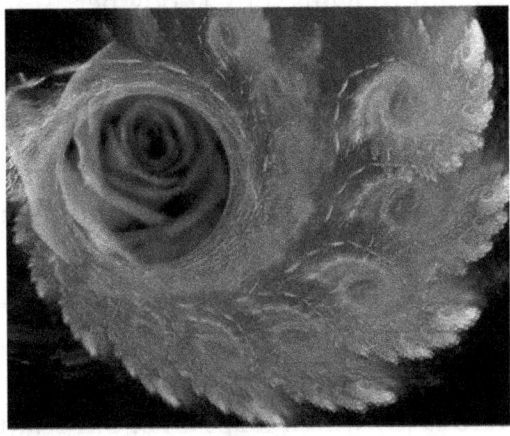

Imagine that you have a close significant other and how you feel about them: (I'll use my ideal vision of a woman as my subject since I'm a guy)

- She makes me happy to be near her
- Her beauty is stunning and I hold her in awe
- She loves the same things I do including places to go, things to do, and foods to eat
- Not being with her makes me feel empty
- She creates joy in me just being there for me.
- I want to hold her close always
- I want to make love to her
- I want to have children with her
- When we fight there is still a background of love
- I want to spend my life with her
- Thinking about life without her is unimaginable
- Losing her from my life would be like cutting off a limb
- Finding out that she has problems or limitations only make me love her
- more since it makes her seem more of a real person

- She is the woman of my dreams
- Being with her makes my heart sing
- We both love God and want to reach oneness

Now if you can imagine a person in your life like the above—then imagine those feelings streaming out of you all of the time for everything in the universe—all living things and everything around you.

Now increase these feelings a hundred fold and imagine that this force of love is what is streaming out of you like a brilliant light.

If you can imagine all this—then maybe you can start to glimpse the full state of Unconditional Love resting in the hands of God—except not directed to a single person—but to everyone and everything around you.

My Heart Opening Experience

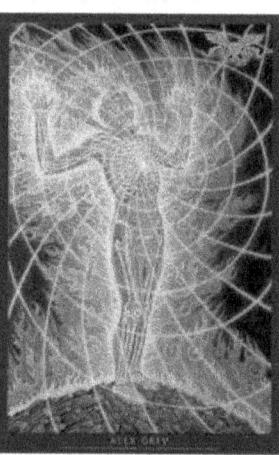

I had previously experienced a few occasional heart openings over the last couple of years from the "Heart Rose" exercise.

My most recent experiences put those previous ones to shame.

In September of 2012 a close female friend of mine who I love dearly told me that she had always loved me unconditionally but not romantically.

Our discussion finally led me to conclude that intimacy was not in our future. However, this woman was someone I had a very deep spiritual connection to and who already had an open heart.

I think spending a lot of time with her over a couple of years plus some other training and experiences of mine had raised my vibrational level to a point where I was ready for a full heart opening.

The process started when I reviewed my feelings for her in my own mind—where my ego was very hurt. Then I recalled all of the good times we had experienced and the spiritual healing and different she had made in my life.

As I reviewed those experiences and realized how grateful I was for them happening was when my heart started to open… in a much greater way than ever before.

There was a lot of heat in my heart and I could feel the heat spreading throughout my body. I also felt more "connected" to everyone and everything than I was before.

This experience went on for hours and happened to some extent everyday thereafter.

I might just be sitting on my couch watching TV and suddenly my heart would open and I would feel wonderful and like my body was being charged with a powerful energy…

Sometimes the energy collecting in my chest gets so powerful that I feel a lot of pressure like a heart attack. I may have to exercise or cool myself off to relieve the pressure. (It's definitely not a medical issue since the pressure quickly goes away and there are no other heart attack symptoms.)

I had learned at the age of nineteen to open my crown chakra and take in energy for healing but this heart experience was an order of magnitude more powerful—and just felt like a different and more personal forms of energy. This experience has become the second major spiritual milestone in my life.

It felt-and still feels today like a drug sometimes where I'm getting high just sitting there and experiencing this natural spiritual life force in my life.

As the last few months have progressed I am beginning to truly understand the spiritual experience that the tongues of fire are described as in the Bible:

ACTS 2:3 And there appeared to them tongues as of fire distributing themselves, and they rested on each one of them.

This is since I was experiencing that fire in my heart—a burning sensation which is pleasurable and doesn't really burn me.

It's kind of like being on a drug—but with only good side effects.

I've also realized that the opening is continuing—it's not a onetime maximum experience but an evolution of the spirit within my body.

Some other effects I've noticed is that people have started treating me differently—especially women. It's like they subconsciously sense the change in my energy and want to get close to me.

Although I'm a fairly attractive middle aged guy I'm not used to beautiful women I don't know starting conversations with me and initiating contact.

I'm also not used to a stranger at a restaurant counter reaching into her purse to change a twenty dollar bill of mine. I didn't ask her to do this—she just looked at me and did it when I asked for change.

Several other experiences come to mind—but you get the idea. Everyone seems to resonate with a person who has an open heart. They sense the spirit of God has come down into that person and want to be closer to it.

This energy of the spirit has also increased my healing ability and has improved my immune system so that I'm not experiencing the colds and flus of my family and the people around me. In previous years I would have caught all of these diseases.

This whole experience has been a great blessing in my life.

****

Now, for the first time in my whole life I truly realize from my experiences with heart opening that my ultimate happiness is inside of me, not in a relationship with somebody.

A relationship can add to the positive aspects of my life, but will not create a happy relationship in itself.

****

I also want to tell you about my emotional effects from the heart opening since I find myself more connected to everyone and everything around me and the "hole" I used to have in my heart is gone.

This "hole" is something I've experience throughout most of my life—even after many years of spiritual development. I always felt that something was empty inside of me.

I'm sure that this "lack" inside of me also affected my relationships—both friends and lovers—for many years.

Now that the emotional "hole" has been filled I feel wonderful and want everyone to be able to enjoy what I've been so blessed to experience.

In talking with other spiritual persons who have experienced heart openings—most of them seem to be women. Maybe it's because women are naturally centered closer to their heart than men. I don't know—but its interesting food for thought.

I do feel that I now have an extra dimension of experience in all types of relationships. The spiritual dimension of love and the connections it creates seems to overlay the emotional and intellectual relationship connections that used to be all I knew.

This spiritual dimension lets me experience other people more fully, and better see the oneness and perfection in all of us.

Additional Research

My additional readings took me to some books on Kundalini including one titled "Kundalini Rising: Exploring the Energy of Awakening" (Khalsa, 2009)

The Kundalini awakening experience most people report has many similarities to the heart opening experience. This makes sense since in Yogic Kundalini traditions it's the Heart Chakra which results in the greatest awakening experiences.

These experiences may happen after many years of meditation and prayer—or just spontaneously- or never.

There is no telling what will happen to the individual. Whether a person's heart opens is a blessing of God's.

Another great book on learning how to use your newly opened heart is titled "Count Your Blessings: The Healing Power of Gratitude and Love" By Dr. John F. Dimartini

This book provides some additional powerful techniques to help people open their hearts through focusing on the positive aspects of all experiences.

Here are some of the main steps to this form of realization:

Choose an experience or condition which has a lot of pain

Then realize that all experiences have positive and negative aspects

Make a list of ten of the positive aspects or lessons learns from the experience.

Finally, give gratitude and thanks to your heart for the positive experience and lessons from this event or condition in your life.

This process of gratitude and thanks needs to be intense and continuous until the participant is brought to tears.

Then the experience can be released and the heart will either open or be brought closer to that wonderful experience.

Summary on Unconditional Love:

Love is more than an abstraction or strong feeling; it is one of the fundamental reasons for living.

From a spiritual perspective the enlightened masters and even the Bible all say that God is Love. That without this force of love in God there would be no Universe.

What could be a more important subject to write about that this?

I know that nothing I've said here is totally unique—since love has been discussed forever.

I just hope I gave you the reader some new food for thought and helped to lighten your day. J

In the next chapter we will look at what your vital forces are and how activating them in your life will also improve your level of energy and long term health.

7.0 Activate Your Vital Forces

The sixth principle of personal longevity is to activate your vital forces.

We all have an energy body which can be represented by concepts of our "human aura", "chakras", and Chinese "energy meridians".

Below is an introduction to some of these concepts and examples of practices you can use to vitalize yourself.

Energy Flows and Chakra Development

The Chinese concept of energy meridians (the points and channels along which energy moves) are used in acupuncture therapy and are another way of looking at the energy flows a body needs.

These and the Indian concept of energy centers (chakras) are all about the way your energy body is designed to stay healthy when energy flows are working properly.

Below is a diagram of the main acupuncture meridians of the body:

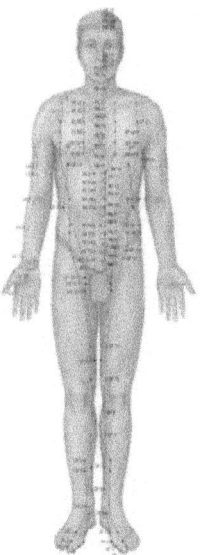

Human Body Acupuncture Meridians

When those flows are interrupted it affects our health and acupuncture can be used to restore this. Needles are used by acupuncturists to stop and start energy moving at key meridian points to help restore the energy body to a proper balance.

Chakra development exercises also help repair energy flows.

In long lived persons the energy is often not flowing properly and has to be repaired. These improvements help one's health; and as the energy starts moving properly again. The energy body is affecting the physical body in a more healthy way.

Many books and traditions discuss details of energy meridians and chakra development so I will not do so here. A short summary of Chakras and their functions follows.

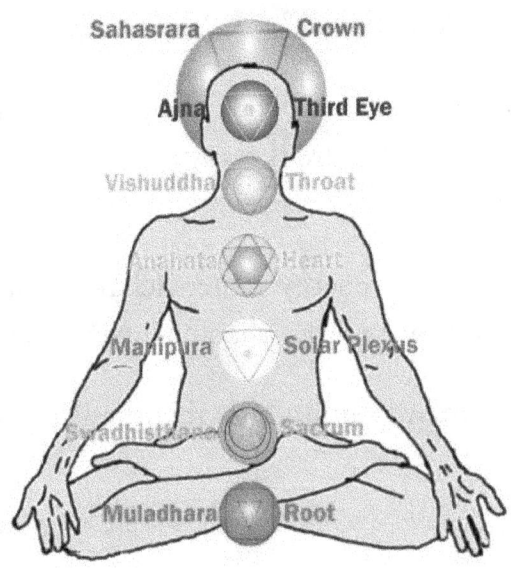

The Figure above shows the chakra centers on the body. These chakras are energy centers where you take in energy to keep your body healthy. The chakras when developed are commonly thought to control spiritual and mental abilities as follows:

<u>Crown Chakra</u>: *To be open, to know, intuition, precognition, connection with infinite intelligence, to have faith and connection with God*

<u>3rd eye Chakra</u>: *Clairvoyance, psychic reading, to have vision or insight, photographic memory and telekinesis*

<u>Throat Chakra</u>: *Communication center, telepathy, clairaudience, inner voice and tone healing*

<u>Heart Chakra</u>: *To be in affinity with, to be at one with, to connect with, compassion and unconditional love*

<u>Solar Plexus Chakra</u>: *Astral projection, to be empowered, to manifest, to be in control of yourself, psychic healing and levitation*

<u>Sacrum/Feeling Chakra</u>: *Clairsentience, emotional feelings, balance of male and female energies*

<u>Root Chakra</u>: *Grounding, realizing, letting go, and surviving*

Meditation is almost always a prerequisite to being able to develop these energy centers.

One example of a positive youthful effect of Chakra development in my life has to do with my head of hair.

I've been developing my crown chakra since I was 18 years old. Now in my fifties, all the men in my family are well on the way to being bald at my age.

However, I still have a full head of hair. I attribute this to the energies which come into my crown chakra daily and which have extended the life of my hair follicles.

The root chakra is where the Kundalini comes from. One must be careful in developing this one since it can cause major imbalances in the others.

It is recommended to find a worthy instructor to develop these energy centers as part of a spiritual development process.

Below is a Crown Chakra Energy Intake Exercise which works well for me.

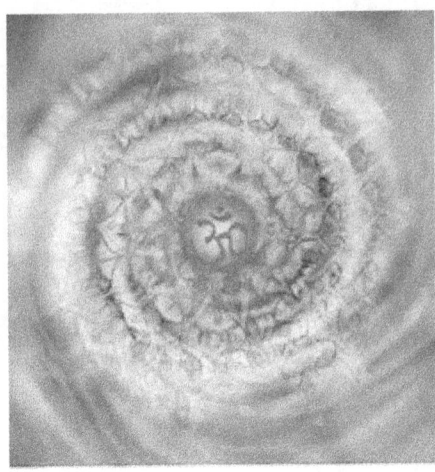

The Crown Chakra or Thousand Petal Lotus

The following exercise on taking in energy through your crown chakra works very well for me and helps energize the energy pathways and chakras in my body. I've used this approach successfully for years.

It may take several times doing this before you start to feel the heat in the top of your head as a result.

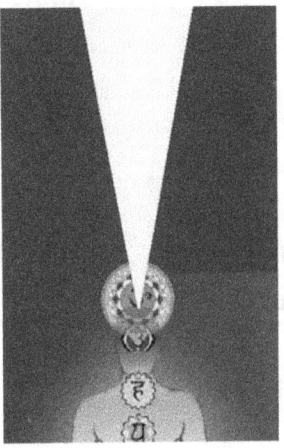

Crown Chakra Energy Intake

Learning to take in Energy through your crown chakra:

Go through a 5-10 minute relaxation exercise while sitting up.

Now visualize a large cone coming from infinity into the top of your head. (See the figure above) It intersects the crown chakra.

Also, visualize your crown chakra as the 1000 petal lotus blossom which is opening as you will it; and as the energy enters your head.

Imagine a large amount of energy and white light is funneling down towards your head, and that as it does so the energy becomes more compressed and more powerful.

The energy enters your head and when it starts to flow you should feel heat in the top of your head; then the energy will flow into your body.

Keep using your will to pump in the energy. First send it to open your third eye to take in energy there too.

Now the energy travels down your neck to open the throat chakra.

Next the energy pours into your chest. When it really gets going it's like a pleasant warmth or fire in your chest. Keep visualizing the energy condensing into the funnel and going into your head and down your body as we continue this exercise.

Next the energy opens your heart and solar plexus chakras. As those open you will feel more energy pouring into your chest; and in the case of the heart chakra—unconditional love.

As the energy travels down your chest it reaches your navel and your sacrum chakra. As it reaches that chakra, again feel it opening and energy pouring into you.

At last the energy reaches your root chakra at the base of the spine. The root chakra also draws fiery energy from beneath the earth. This energy is called kundalini.

Now imagine that your root chakra is anchored into the ground; and this kundalini fire will pass upwards through your spine. You feel the fire coursing up your spine and eventually into your head.

Now you have the full flow of energies throughout the major chakras of your body. Keep visualizing the energy coming in through your crown and circulating down to the root; and then the kundalini circling back up. As this happens it opens all your energy centers more and you will feel the energy pouring into you. (Do this for five more minutes)

Practices and Exercises for your Body

The ideas behind the exercises mentioned in this chapter are that all of them work on the body's vital force to make sure the "CHI" is flowing correctly in an older body the way it does in a youthful and healthy person.

What is the vital force? It is the force that many traditions believe is the life force, chi, prana, or by any other name—the force of life which animates our physical bodies.

I'm sure there are more types of CHI or Vital Force exercises than I'm aware of. I'm only illustrating several types below.

One should consider finding a teacher of these exercises to help them learn them better.

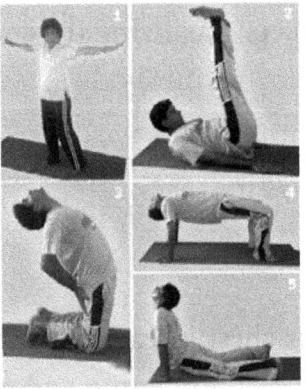

The Five Tibetan Rites

Pictures of The Five Tibetan Rites

These are exercises which should strengthen the body and make it more youthful. I tried them for a year and they do seem to have a positive effect. The original book on this is called "The Eye of Revelation" by Peter Kelder and was first published in 1939. The updated version of this book is called "Ancient Secret of the Fountain of Youth"

In the book the Author recounted a British Colonel's story of how the Colonel lived at a monestary with monks much older tham himslef and how the rites helped rejuvinate him from old age to a vital and younger self.

In the original "The Eye of Revelation" booklet, Kelder never mentions the practice of any type of breathing exercise while performing the first Five Rites.

However, subsequent publications pertaining to the Rites contain edits by others which recommend and detail specific instructions for breathing while performing the exercises. Some practitioners also recommend taking caution prior to performing the Rites due to the possibility of aggravating certain health conditions.

Kelder cautions that when performing the First Rite, spinning must always be performed in a *clockwise* direction. He also states that Bradford clearly recalled that the aulawiyah, otherwise known as "Whirling Dervishes", always spun from left to right, in a clockwise direction. No mention is made of the positioning of the palms, although the original illustration of the Rite in the 1939 edition of *"The Eye of Revelation"* clearly depicts both palms as facing downwards towards the ground.

First Rite - Clockwise Whirling Inhale and exhale deeply as you spin.

Second Rite - Head and Leg Raises Inhale deeply while lifting the head and legs, exhale while lowering the head and legs.

Third Rite – Camel Inhale as the spine arches back, exhale as the spine returns to an erect position.

Fourth Rite – Tabletop Inhale while rising up, hold the breath while in the top position and tense the muscles, then exhale while returning to the starting position.

Fifth Rite - Up and Down Dog Inhale while raising the body, exhale while lowering the body. Sixth Rite - (Uddiyana Bandha Abdominal Breathing Exercise)

Claimed benefits of performing the rites:

According to Kelder, Bradford's stay in the lamasery transformed him from a stooped, old gentleman with a cane to a tall and straight young man in the prime of his life.

Additionally, he reported that Bradford's hair had grown back and without a trace of gray.

The revised publishing's of *The Eye of Revelation* entitled *Ancient Secret of the Fountain of Youth* also contain numerous testimonials by practitioners of the Rites claiming that they yield positive medical effects such as improved eyesight, memory, potency, hair growth, restoring full color to completely gray hair and anti-aging.

The benefits most likely to be achieved are increased energy, stress reduction and an enhanced sense of calm, clarity of thought, increased strength & flexibility and an overall improvement in health and well-being.

Seamm Jasani or Gentle Boabom (58 Movements for Eternal Youth)

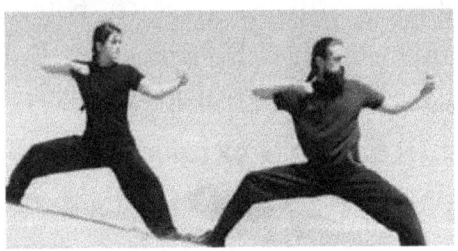

Seamm Jasani Exercises

Seamm Jasani or Gentle Boabom is a system of moving meditation, active relaxation, and self-defense. Teachers stress while the movements learned in the art could effectively be used in combat situations, the central aim of the practice is to heighten bodily awareness and help the student attain an optimal state of health, energy, and vitality.

The exercises involve bodily movements which increase the flow of vital forces in your body. The Art is developed through:

The Path of Gentle Movement, and
The Path of Union: Movement Breathing, Mind

The Path of Gentle Movement is based on controlled psychical physical movements and forces the muscles, nerves and brain to work in a manner completely outside of the routine that they are used to.

In the Path of Union-The coordinations that are developed here vary and form a dance, or active meditation, as body, breathing, mind and imagination are all working together simultaneously.

The results of these movements are the following:

- Tranquility
- Energy
- Happiness and
- great positivity

that can be used in any way the student wants, for personal, professional, or student needs. It is an energy recharger.

Qigong Teachings

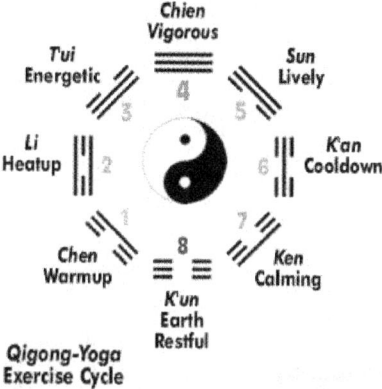

Qigong is a set of exercises related to Tai Chi. It is just now becoming known in the Western world.

In the book "Qigong Teachings of a Taoist Immortal" the Author refers to three ways a person can use the Tao in their quest for immortality:

Herbal medicines and dietary regimes Physical and respiratory exercises

The third is the achievement of mental and physical tranquility.

Qi is the "breath" or "vital energy" which Qigong exercises seek to move throughout the body. The Qi (CHI) is contained within meridians (energy pathways) in the body.

Through the stimulation and accumulation of qi a person may not only acquire a new sense of physical and mental energy, but create the conditions of longevity as well.

In order to fully mobilize the Qi throughout the body one must first accumulate it in what is the called the tan-t'ien (Field of Elixer). This tan-t'tien is a point in the lower abdomen about three inches below the navel and one inch back into the body.

When one learns to accomplish nine complete circulations in one sitting then immortality is achieved and what is produced is called the "immortal fetus" or "qi body".

There are also a variety of physical exercises one can do in QiGong which help strengthen the energy flows in the body and result in better health. These are best learned from a Master teaching the techniques.

In the classes I take, Qi Gong exercises are used to loosen up and start the vital force flowing before starting the Tai Chi forms.

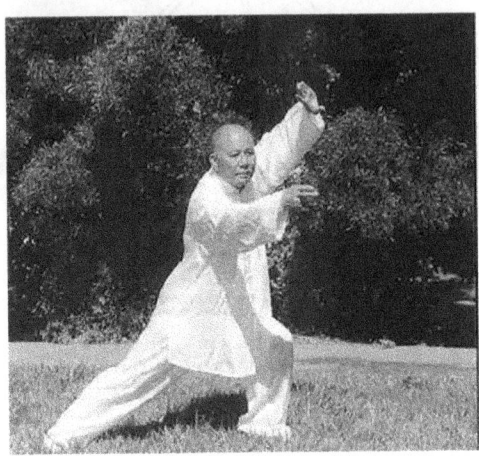

Tai Chi Chuan

Tai Chi Chuan is practiced by millions of Chinese and is now becoming popular in the West.

Tai chi chuan is typically practiced for a variety of reasons: its soft martial techniques, demonstration competitions, health and longevity. Consequently, a multitude of training forms exist, both traditional and modern, which correspond to those aims. Some of tai chi chuan's training forms are well known to Westerners as the slow motion routines that groups of people practice together every morning indoors and outdoors around the world, particularly in China.

Most modern styles of Tai chi trace their development to at least one of the five traditional schools: Chen, Yang, Wu/Hao, Wu and Sun. The origins and creation of tai chi is a subject of much argument and speculation. However, the oldest documented tradition is that of the Chen family from the 1820s.

The study of Tai Chi Chuan primarily involves three aspects:

Health: An unhealthy, or otherwise uncomfortable person, may find it difficult to meditate to a state of calmness or to use tai chi as a martial art. Tai chi's health training therefore concentrates on relieving the physical effects of stress on the body and mind. For those focused on Tai Chi's martial arts, good physical fitness is an important step towards effective self-defense.

Meditation: The focus and calmness cultivated by the meditative aspect of Tai Chi is seen as necessary in relieving stress and maintaining homeostasis and in application of the form as a soft style martial art.

Martial art: The ability to use Tai Chi as a form of self-defense in combat is the test of a student's understanding of the art. Tai Chi Chuan martially is the study of appropriate change in response to outside forces; the study of yielding and "sticking" to an incoming attack rather than attempting to meet it with opposing force.

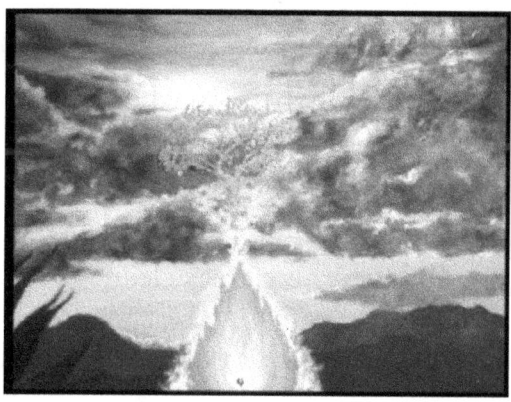

Sacred Fire Visualizations

There are a variety of visualization techniques which can also help heal and make your body more vibrant.

One of these is the Sacred Fire visualization. (Also known as the Violet Flame). The technique relies on first putting yourself into a deep meditative trance.

Then you visualize that you are inside a pillar of white fire which penetrates every cell of your being. That the pillar extends out to six feet from you.

Center yourself in the center of your head at the pineal gland. The traditional location of the spirit or soul in the body.

Imagine a bright light there like a flame. This light is getting brighter and expanding. This white light is the light of the spirit and the power of God.

The light expands to fill your head then travels down your neck into your chest. Imagine that the light starts to fill you with purity and health.

The bright white light travels down your body, into your arms, the rest of your torso, and into your legs. This goes on until your body is a vessel of white light.

Now the light expands outward from the surface of your body. It's now expanded to a few inches outside your body.

Then the light expands further, out to five feet, then ten feet so that you are the center of a sphere of light and consciousness.

Feel this power becoming more intense within and outside of your body.

Now start in your head and see the light washing away any impurities in your head, that any unhealthy or diseased cells are being washed away and will be expelled from the body.

As you move down your body examining yourself mentally you may see some areas which are dark. The light will burn these areas clean.

In addition you know that this infinite spirit of God is immortalizing your body, bit by bit.

As your senses travel down your body the dark areas you sense are washed pure and the cells in those places are immortalized.

Do this for your entire body.

You are at the center of the sphere of light and your body has been purified and immortalized down to the smallest cells during this process.

Imagine that this Fire is anchored in and around you and will be constantly working until you have achieved Ascension.

You should do this every day after meditating to get to a very relaxed state.

The books "Unveiled Mysteries" and "The Magic Presence" are suggested to readers to learn more about the Violet Flame as it was related to the author by the Immortal and Ascended Master Count St. Germain.

Cellular Regeneration

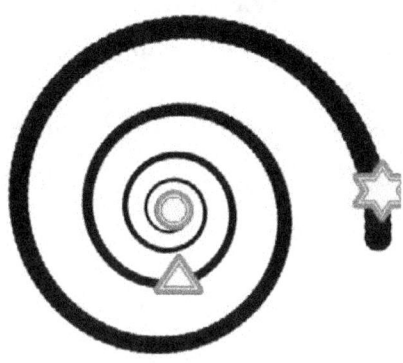

The Reverse Spiral of Aging

The concept of cellular regeneration is one in which we use the power of visualization to command our cells to reverse their age to an earlier one.

In other words, this is a method of making your body younger by learning how to "youth" the cells in your body.

The following technique also has an interesting side effect. The effect was described that after a person has been using this technique for a while they or others may smell "old shoe smell" coming from themselves as the body's cells start to get rid of toxins. (You can remove the smell by taking a shower).

The morning after my first session doing this exercise—which was a really intense one—my son complained that I smelled like old shoes—and he had never complained about my smell before.

The exercise follows:

The spiral picture above has circle for the beginning of cell's life, a star for the current state, and triangle for the age you want to revert to. The spiral is counter clockwise to represent going back in time

Go through a relaxation procedure for 5-10 minutes:

Choose the age you would like your cells to revert to. Is it 20 years old, or 29?, or another age. Pick an age that you would like your body to be as an immortal.

Visualize that you have microscopic vision and can see into the cells in your left foot. They are at the same size as in the movie "The Fantastic Voyage". You can move your attention between thousands of cells and recognize the cell's age in each case.

Now start visualizing that you feel your consciousness inside the entire foot where you can see millions of cells; and that the cells have a level of consciousness too. Then tell them all to revert to your chosen age.

Now you see tiny counterclockwise spirals inside each cell as each one follows your direction to start reverting to a younger age.

You feel an energy in your left foot that is tingly like electricity as the cells start the reversion process.

Now start imagining a counter clockwise spiral outside of your foot centered on your foot and moving up your leg slowly. As it moves up your leg each cell is also taking conscious direction and starts its own reverse spiral to revert to your target age.

The spiral moves up to the top of your leg; and as it does the cells within, down to the bone and bone marrow, start their counter clockwise age reversion. Your cells are conscious and part of you so they take direction from you.

Do the same thing in the other leg, then moving up the torso, then the arms, and finally the neck and head. Do each part slowly, and keep emphasizing the microscopic cells with tiny spirals reverting as well as the macroscopic spiral spinning around the part of the body you are working on.

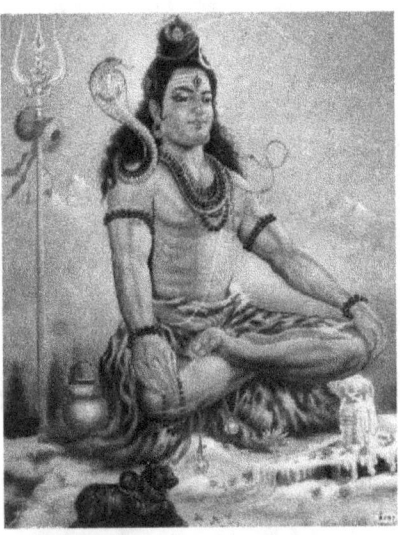

Hatha Yoga Breathing Exercises

The following exercises to promote health and immortality are from an online copy of a book Titled "Relax with Yoga" originally authored by Arthur Liebers in 1960.

This information provides an excellent overview of Hatha Yoga breathing exercises, and discusses the results which should be expected according to ancient Yogic writings. (the Yoga Sutras of Patanjali

Among the "secret" aspects of Yoga are the Bandhas. After the body has been prepared by thorough practice in the different *asanas* and clarified by preliminary breathing exercises, the Yogi is ready for the Bandhas. These may not be attained immediately, since they depend on a full state of physical and mental relaxation for successful attainment.

The Mudras:

According to Hindu sages, the ten *mudras* destroy old age and death, having been given out by the God Shiva, and also confer the eight *siddhis* or miraculous powers. The old text enjoins the student to secrecy, saying, "This should be carefully kept secret as a box of diamonds and should not be told to anybody—just as the illicit connection with a married woman of noble family." Descriptions of the ten *mudras* follow.

Jalandhara Bandha

Get into a comfortable siddhasana or sukhasana cross-legged seated position with the palms facing down on top of the knees. Let the spine be long, the shoulders relaxed down and the sternum lifted. Let the eyes softly close and the breath slow and deepen. Take a slow deep inhale to two thirds of your lung's capacity and hold the breath in. Drop the chin to the chest and draw it in so the back of the neck stays long and does not round. Let the shoulders roll very slightly forward to deepen the lock in the throat, but keep them soft.

Maha Mudra

Pressing the anus with the left heel and stretching the left leg, take hold of the toes with your hand. Then practice the Jalandhara Bandha (described above), and draw your breath through the *susumna* (the space behind the navel). Then the *kundalini* (the sleeping goddess within the internal organs) becomes straight, just as a coiled snake does when struck, and the *ida* (left nostril) and *pingala* (right nostril) become dead, because the breath goes out of them. The breath should be let out slowly, never quickly.

Maha Bandha

Having restrained your breath as long as possible, breathe out slowly. Practice first on the left side, then on the right. This is said to stop the upward course of the breath through the *nadis* (nerves) except the *susumna* (spinal cord), and brings about the union of them with the *susumna* and enable the mind to remain fixed between the two eyebrows. The above two *mudras* are described as having limited value without a third, called the Maha Vedha.

Maha Vedha

Draw in your breath with a concentrated mind and stop the upward and downward course of breath by the Jalandhara Bandha. Sitting on the ground with your body on your hands, gently seat and raise yourself repeatedly. Then breathe out. The body assumes a deathlike aspect in this exercise.

Kechari Mudra

This is not likely to appeal to the Westerner seeking beneficial aspects of Yoga. This *mudra* requires the following preparation: By slight daily cutting, continued for six months, the ligament which holds down the tongue is severed. By repeated pulling, the tongue is made long enough to reach the eyebrows. The *mudra* is performed by turning the tongue up and in, so that it enters the hole in the palate where the three *nadis* (nerves) join. Simultaneously, the eyes should be fixed firmly between the brows. (The author is not recommending this technique.)

Vajroli Mudra

Said to give five Siddhis, even to one who lives an ordinary life, along with the *amaroli* and *sahajoli*, which are linked with it, this *mudra* occupies another 20 *sutras*, or verses, which are almost impossible to translate into English because of their mystic character. The commentary on the Sanskrit text says that they are not to be understood literally. Further, they are incomplete in some points which are left to be filled by verbal instructions from the *guru*, or Yoga teacher or leader.

Shakati Chalana

Named as the last of the ten mudras, this is described as follows: Having inhaled through the right nostril, the practitioner should retain his breath and "manipulate the kundalini for about an hour and a half, both at morning and evening twilights."

The Sanskrit text states:

"As one forces open the door with a key, so should the Yogi force open the door of *moksha* (state of bliss) by the *kundalini*. The *kundalini* gives *mukti* (deliverance) to the Yogis and bondage to the fools. He who knows her, knows Yoga. He who causes that *shakti* (the *kundalini*) to move (from the *muladhara* in the pelvic region upwards) is freed without doubt. Between the *ganges* (*ida*) and *jamuna* (*pingala*) there sits the young widow inspiring pity. He (the Yogi) should despoil her forcibly, for it leads one to the supreme seat of Vishnu. You should awaken the sleeping serpent (*kundalini*) by taking hold of its tail. Seated in the *vajrasena* posture, firmly take hold of the ankle and slowly beat with them the *kanda* [something below the navel from which the 72,000 *nadis* issue].

By moving the *kundalini* fearlessly for about an hour and a half, she is drawn upwards a little through the *susumna*," which process, it is claimed, "surely opens the mouth of the *susumna* and the breath naturally goes through it." Whether this effect is produced by manipulation of the *kundalini* or other means, it seems to be the object primarily aimed at in Hatha Yoga practice. The fruits of the practice of Hatha Yoga, taken in the order of their mention in the texts, are:

1. The eight *siddhis*: *anima* (the power to assimilate oneself with an atom); *mahima* (the power to expand oneself into space); *laghima* (the power to be as light as cotton or any similar thing); *garima* (the power to be as heavy as anything); *prapti* (the power of reaching anywhere, even to the moon); *prakamya* (the power of having all wishes, of whatever description, realized); *isvata* (power to create); *vasvita* (power to command all).
2. Freedom from death and old age.
3. Rejuvenation and perpetual youth.
4. Beauty.
5. Ability to "do and undo."
6. Exemption from hunger, thirst and indolence.

7. Ability to walk on water.
8. Attainment of anything in the three worlds.
9. Invulnerability of wrinkles and gray hair.
10. Removal of wrinkles and gray hair.
11. Freedom from disease.
12. Exemption from the effects of Karma.
13. Immortality and the eight *siddhis* named above.
14. Power to attract the other sex.

The above 14 siddhis are implied by powers mentioned in "The Yoga Sutras of Patanjali" (25)

Finally, and beyond the *siddhis*, comes the grand result of *mukti*, or emancipation from rebirth, and the conscious junction with Brahman. These powers are certainly all that could be desired; in fact, they stop nothing short of omnipotence, omnipresence and omniscience, but we must allow for the ever-pervading Eastern hyperbole, and for the mystical superstructure of the ancient Hindu school of physiology.

Chapter Summary

As you have read in this chapter, there are many types of practices to help increase the flow and intensity of vital forces in your body.

There are also many more practices than those described in this chapter.

I encourage you to seek our those practices and determine which are the best for you, then do it!

In the next chapter we get into different types of science and research on aging with some practical advice which you can use to improve your body's health.

8.0 The Science of Longevity

The seventh principle of personal longevity is to utilize current medical and scientific research on longevity.

Since the 10 principles are intended to utilize both unconventional holistic approaches and long term and current scientific and medical practices, we would be remiss if we didn't discuss the latest medical and scientific research and practices.

Long Lived Plants and Animals

One of the reasons to look at long lived plants and animals is because they have a similar genetic make-up and heritage to ourselves. If these plants and animals can have such long lives we can see what the potential physical limits are in our own physical bodies.

Clonal colonies

As with all long-lived plants and fungal species, no individual part of a clonal colony is alive (in the sense of active metabolism) for more than a very small fraction of the life of the entire clone. Some clonal colonies may be fully connected via their root systems; while most are not actually interconnected, but are genetically identical clones which populate an area through vegetative reproduction. Ages for clonal colonies, often based on current growth rates, are estimates:

A huge colony of the sea grass *Posidonia Oceanica* in the Mediterranean Sea could be up to 100,000 years old.

Pando (tree). This clonal colony of *Populus Tremuloides* has been estimated at 80,000 years old, although some claims place it as being as old as one million years.

King's Lomatia in Tasmania: The sole surviving clonal colony of this species is estimated to be at least 43,600 years old.

A huckleberry bush in Pennsylvania is thought to be as much as 13,000 years old.

Eucalyptus Recurva: Clones in Australia are claimed to be 13,000 years old.

Creosote bush: A ring of bushes in the Mojave Desert are estimated at 11,700 years of age.

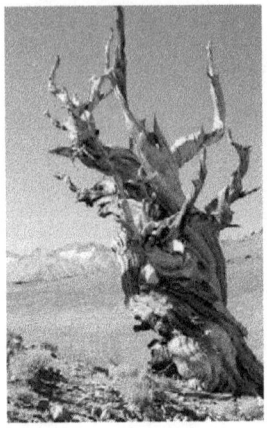

Methuselah-The World's Oldest Tree at 4,838 years old

An individual of the fungus species *Armillaria Ostoyae* in the Malheur National Forest is thought to be between 2,000 and 8,500 years old. It is thought to be the world's largest organism by area, at 2,384 acres (965 hectares).

Individual plant specimens

A cluster of Norway spruce in Sweden includes roots that have been carbon dated to 9,550 years old, which would make them the oldest known trees in the world! Individual tree trunks only last up to about 600 years, but the roots from which they grow have survived throughout the entire period.

A Great Basin Bristlecone Pine (*Pinus Longaeva*) called Prometheus was measured by ring count at 4,862 years old when it was felled in 1964. This is the greatest verified age for any living organism at this time. Another great basin Bristlecone Pine, known as Methuselah, measured by ring count of sample cores is, at 4,838 years old, the oldest known tree in North America, and the oldest known individual tree in the world.

Fortingall Yew, an ancient yew (Taxus Baccata) in the churchyard of the village of Fortingall in Perthshire, Scotland; is possibly the oldest known individual tree in Europe. Various estimates have put its age at between 2000 and 5000 years.

Fitzroya Cupressoides is the species with the second oldest verified age, a specimen in Chile being measured by ring count as 3,622 years old.

A Sacred Fig (*Ficus Religiosa*) specimen, the Sri Maha Bodhi, is (if its reported planting date of 288 BC is correct) at 2,293 years old, is the oldest known flowering plant.

A specimen of <u>*Lagarostrobos Franklinii*</u> in Tasmania is thought to be about 2000 years old.

Numerous Olive trees are purported to be 2000 years old or older. An olive tree in Crete, claiming such longevity, has been confirmed on the basis of tree ring analysis.

<u>Animals</u>

The Hydrozoan species *Turritopsis nutricula* is capable of cycling from a mature adult stage to an immature polyp stage and back again, indefinitely. This means there is, theoretically, no limit to its life span. Although no single specimen has been observed for any extended period and it is impossible to estimate the age of a specimen.

The Antarctic sponge *Cinachyra Antarctica* has an extremely slow growth rate in the low temperatures of the Antarctic Ocean. One specimen has been estimated to be 1,550 years old.

A specimen of the Icelandic Cyprine *Arctica Islandica* (also known as an ocean Quahog), a mollusk, was found to have lived 405 years and possibly up to 410. Another specimen had a recorded lifespan of 374 years.

Some Koi fish have reportedly lived up to over 200 years, the oldest being Hanko; which died at an age of 215 years on July 7, 1977.

Some unconfirmed sources estimated Bowhead whales to have lived up to 210 years of age. If proven this would make them the oldest mammals.

Specimens of the Red Sea Urchin, Strongylocentrotus Franciscanus, have been found to be over 200 years old.

Tu'i Malila, a radiated tortoise, died at an age of 188 years in May 1965. Harriet, a Galápagos tortoise died at an unconfirmed age of 175 years in June 2006.

Timothy, a Greek tortoise, died at an age of 160 years in April 2004.

Geoduck, a species of saltwater clam native to the Puget Sound, have been known to live over 160 years.

A 109-year old female Blue-and-yellow Macaw named Charlie was hatched in 1899. It was incorrectly claimed that she formerly belonged to Winston Churchill.

There is anecdotal evidence that the Patagonian tooth fish and sturgeon can live for over 100 years.

The deep-sea hydrocarbon seep tubeworm *Lamellibrachia Luymesi* (Annelida, Polychaeta) lives for over 170 years.

The Ocean Quahog (a clam) has been found to have specimans as old as 405 years. There are numerous other animals that live to more than 200 years.

What current science says about longevity

a. The increase in Life Expectancy

Life expectancy is the average number of years a human has before death. It is conventionally calculated from the time of birth, but also can be calculated from any specified age.

Advances in sanitation, nutrition, and medical knowledge have made possible incredible changes in life expectancy throughout the world; providing subjects for study as well as the need to study them. In the United States, only 50 percent of children born in 1900 were expected to reach the age of 50; life expectancy today is approximately 83 years of age. But note that there is a significant difference between male and female life expectancy - 82 years for men and 85 years for women. Life expectancy is lower for African Americans; 67.2 years for men and 74.7 years for women (Hoyert, Kochanek, and Murphy, 1999).

Life expectancy increased dramatically in the 20th century. These changes are the result of a combination of factors including nutrition, public health, and medicine only marginally. The most important single factor in the increase is the reduction of death in infancy.

The greatest improvements have been in the richest parts of the world. Life expectancy at birth in the United States in 1900 was 47 years. Life expectancy in India at mid-century was around 32, by 2000 it had risen to 64 years. According to the 2006 World Health Organization Report, due to HIV/AIDS and other health related issues today's life expectancy in poorer nations is almost half that of the industrialized, richer nations.

You will be able to see in the table below that for most of human history life expectancy was only 20- 30 years old. What we would now consider young adulthood.

It was only in the early 20th Century that the average length of life went up to 40 years.

The number of today's Octogenarians would be considered amazing and mostly unbelievable to people living 100 years ago.

Totay's average world life expectancy of 66 years seems low to many of us raised in Western Countries.

Is it really that much more far fetched to be discussing how to double our present lifespans from today, considering that they have been doubled in the last 100 years?

The below Table shows how general life expectancy has changed in the world over millennia:

Humans by Era	Average Lifespan at Birth (years)
Neanderthal	20
Upper Paleolithic	33
Neolithic	20
Bronze Age[6]	18
Classical Greece[7]	20-30
Classical Rome[8][9]	20-30
Pre-Columbian North America[10]	25-35
Medieval Britain[11][12]	20-30
Early 20th Century[13][14]	30-40
Current world average[15][16]	66.12 (2008 est.)

Current Life Expectancies Around the World

Here in colors are Life Expectancies over Historical Time Periods with a key for the colors following:

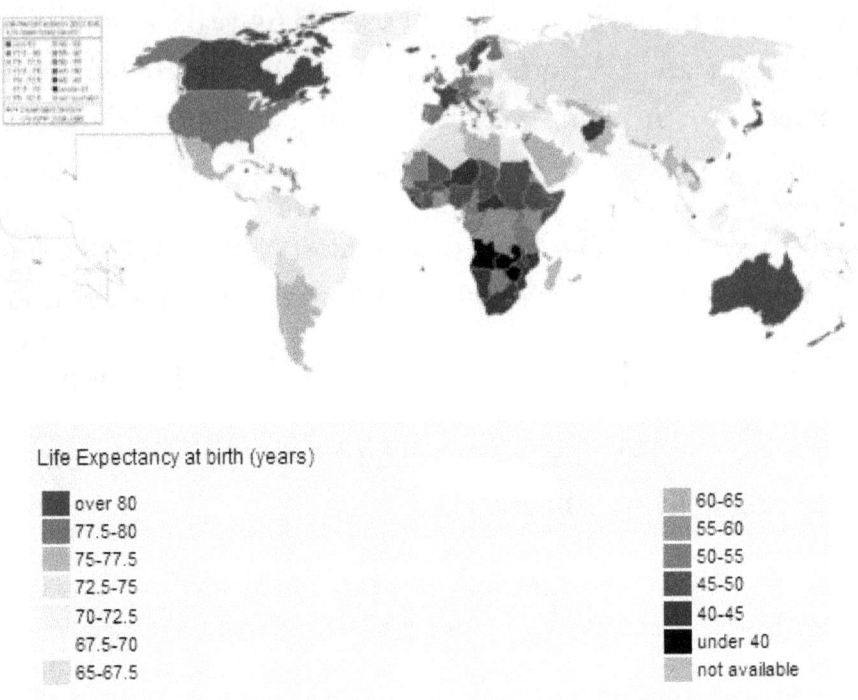

Much work is being done in Science today which may end up increasing our life expectancy significantly.

Below are some of the types of biological immortality science is researching.

Biological Immortality

This can be defined as the absence of a sustained increase in rate of mortality as a function of chronological age. A cell or organism that does not experience, aging, is biologically immortal. However this definition of immortality was challenged in the "Handbook of the Biology of Aging", because the increase in rate of mortality as a function of chronological age may be negligible at extremely old ages (late-life mortality plateau). But even though the rate of mortality ceases to increase in old age, those rates are very high (e.g., 50% chance of surviving another year at age 110 or 115 years of age).

There is no known organism or individual cell that is inviolably immortal. Any life enjoying *biological immortality* can die if exposed to a toxic environment, or otherwise killed or destroyed.

Cell lines

Biologists have chosen the word immortal to designate cells that are not limited by the Hayflick limit (where cells no longer divide because of DNA damage or shortened telomeres). Prior to the work of Leonard Hayflick there was the erroneous belief fostered by Alexis Carrel that all normal somatic cells are immortal.

The term immortalization was first applied to cancer cells that expressed the telomere lengthening enzyme telomerase, and thereby avoided apoptosis (programmed cell death). Among the most commonly used cell lines are HeLa and Jurkat, both of which are immortalized cancer cells. Normal stem cells and germ cells can also be said to be immortal.

Immortal cell lines of cancer cells can be created by induction of oncogenes or loss of tumor suppressor genes. One way to induce immortality is through viral-mediated induction of the large T- antigen, commonly introduced through simian virus 40 (.

In terms of multi-cellular organisms, immortality may not be a desirable condition, as the main controls over cancer are the apoptotic mechanisms.

Bacteria:

Bacteria can be said to be biologically immortal, but only as a colony. An individual bacterium can easily die. The two daughter bacteria resulting from cell division of a parent bacterium can be regarded as unique individuals or as embers of a biologically "immortal" colony. The two daughter cells can be regarded as "rejuvenated" copies of the parent cell because damaged macromolecules have been split between the two cells and diluted. In the same way stem cells and gametes can be regarded as "immortal".

Hydra:

Hydras are a genus of simple, fresh-water animals possessing radial symmetry and no post-mitotic cells. The fact that all cells continually divide allows defects and toxins to be "diluted-away". It has been suggested that hydras do not undergo senescence (aging), and so are biologically immortal.

The FoxO gene has recently been found to make Hydra's immortal and the same gene exists in humans.

Life Extensionists:

Some life extensionists, such as those who practice cryonics, have the hope that humans may someday become biologically immortal. This would not be the same as literal immortality, since people can always be murdered or die in accidents. (Mind uploading, however, could allow literal immortality in a sense, by uploading backups into cloned or artificial bodies after an accident. See Mind uploading in science fiction.) However, this practice may not actually allow for one to continue

their life through the backup, and since two (or more) beings with identical minds have never existed before, it is unknown whether or not they could share consciousness on any level.

Nanotechnology, and specifically of nano-medicine, have recently increased awareness of the possibilities for biological immortality in humans. A study published in Physiological and Biochemical Zoology in 2005 indicates that biological immortality may exist in humans at a late stage in life: "the exponential increase in age-specific death rate seemed to slow down.

Red Wine Extract- Resvesterol

In 2006, Italian scientists obtained the first positive results of resveratrol supplementation in a vertebrate. Using a short-lived fish, *Nothobranchius Furzeri*, with a median life span of nine weeks, they found that a maximal dose of resveratrol increased the median lifespan by 56%. Compared with the control fish at nine weeks, that is by the end of the latter's life, the fish supplemented with resveratrol showed significantly higher general swimming activity and better learning to avoid an unpleasant stimulus. The authors noted a slight increase of mortality in young fish caused by resveratrol, and hypothesized that it is its weak toxic action that stimulated the defense mechanisms and resulted in the life span extension.

Resveratrol is sold as a dietary supplement. See in Herbs Chapter.

Calorie Restriction Diets

In human subjects, CR has been shown to lower cholesterol, fasting glucose, and blood pressure. Some consider these to be biomarkers of aging, since there is a correlation between these markers and risk of diseases associated with aging. Except for houseflies, animal species tested with CR so far, including primates, rats, mice, spiders, *Drosophila*, *C. Elegans* and rotifers, have shown lifespan extension. CR is the only known dietary measure capable of extending maximum lifespan, as opposed to average lifespan. In CR, energy intake is minimized, but sufficient quantities of vitamins, minerals and other important nutrients must be eaten.

In the US at the Washington University School of Medicine in St. Louis a small scale study showing the effects of following a calorie restricted diet of 10-25% less calorie intake than the average Western diet. Body mass index (BMI) was significantly lower in the calorie-restricted group when compared with the matched group; 19.6 compared with 25.9. The BMI values for the comparison group are similar to the mean BMI values for middle-aged people in the US.

Telomeres

A telomere is a region of repetitive DNA at the end of chromosomes, which protects the end of the chromosome from destruction. Its name is derived from the Greek nouns telos (τέλος) "end" and meros (μέρος, root: μερεσ-) "part".

During cell division, the enzymes that duplicate the chromosome and its DNA can't continue their duplication all the way to the end of the chromosome. If cells divided without telomeres, they would lose the end of their chromosomes, and the necessary information it contains. (In 1972, James Watson named this phenomenon the "end replication problem".) The telomere is a disposable buffer, which is consumed during cell division and is replenished by an enzyme, the telomerase reverse transcriptase.

In 1975-1977, Elizabeth Blackburn, working as a postdoctoral fellow at Yale University with Joseph Gall, discovered the unusual nature of telomeres, with their simple repeated DNA sequences composing chromosome ends. Their work was published in 1978.

This mechanism usually limits cells to a fixed number of divisions, and animal studies suggest that this is responsible for aging on the cellular level and affects lifespan.

Telomeres protect a cell's chromosomes from fusing with each other or rearranging. These chromosome abnormalities can lead to cancer, so cells are normally destroyed when telomeres are consumed. Most cancer is the result of cells bypassing the Telomere destruction. Biologists speculate that this mechanism is a tradeoff between aging and cancer.

Some scientists think that by finding a way to lengthen the telomeres in our cells we wouldn't have as much cell damage when cells replicate, and therefore live much longer lives.

There are now supplements on the market which claim to increase the length of telomeres which therefore will lengthen a cell's lifetime.

Electronic, Digital, and Technological Solutions

One area of life extension I'm not addressing in this book is what you might call the technological solution.

These are solutions to download consciousness into computers or provide backup computing power to manage consciousness and memories.

My problem with this approach is that since I strongly believe that all of us have an immortal soul which is separate from our physical bodies. Therefore, any type of currently envisioned technological storage approach would only store a portion of the physical mind-not any elements of the Spirit.

Chapter Summary:

Current research shows us what new things we can being doing to increase our lifespans such as using red wine supplements, calorie restriction diets, or taking telomere enhancing supplements.

In the next chapter we will look at what additional supplements we can take to improve our physical body's health.

9.0 Keep your Physical Body Healthy

The eighth principle of personal longevity is to keep your physical body healthy.

You can't be overweight, eat bad foods, be a couch potato, smoke, or do other unhealthy practices and expect to live a long time.

(In fact one physical trainer I know has said that he never met a person over eighty who weighed more than 250 pounds.)

Since there are thousands of books and professionals who work on diet, exercise, and other bodily health issues, I'm not going to try to repeat what they do.

This Chapter is divided into two parts:

Section A covers mainly herbs and supplements which can be taken to prolong your life. Also some information on the important benefits of regular exercise

Section B covers the Diets and Lifestyles of the World's Oldest Persons.

Section A: Longevity Herbs and Supplements

There are many books in China on Herbalism and how various herbs can increase your long term health and longevity.

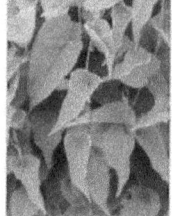

One of my favorite modern books is "The Ancient Wisdom of the Chinese Tonic Herbs" By Ron Teeguarden.

Ron's book explains many of the uses of longevity herbs and different types of herbs and combinations of herbs that people use.

Herbs and Foods

The below herbs are claimed to help with life extension. LI CHING-YUN made Fo-ti-tieng and Ginseng the most popular since he said he took them as teas every day.

Resveratrol has become popular in recent years as studies have shown the health effects of red wine extract.

Not being a medical professional I make no claims about the effectiveness of these herbs—although I do use them myself.

I also do not claim this is an exclusive list of herbs to improve health and lengthen life. There may be many others which also help your body remain young.

Fo-ti-tieng

-Fo-ti-ieng Leaves

History: Was first popularized by long lived Person LI CHING-YUN who said he took it in Tea everyday to help his health

Family Name: Polygonaceae

Botanical Name(s): Polygonum Multiflorum Popular Name(s): He-Shou-Wu, Fo-Ti Parts Used: Unprocessed root

Habitat: Native to China

Uses: The whole root has been used to lower cholesterol levels as well as to decrease hardening of the arteries, or arteriosclerosis. Other fo-ti research has investigated this herb's role in strong immune function, red blood cell formation, and antibacterial action.

Ginseng

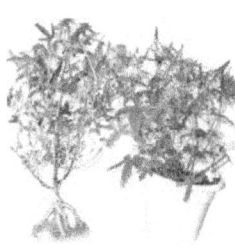

History: Known from ancient times in China to be a general supplement to health and long life. Is believed by some Chinese

Herbalists to help change your body's energy flows back to a healthful state. The thread among centurions is to only use supplements labeled "Panax Ginseng".

Family Name: Araliaceae

Botanical Name(s): Panax Ginseng

Popular Name(s): Ginseng, Asian Asiatic Ginseng, Chinese Ginseng, Asian Ginseng

Parts Used: Root

Habitat: It grows in the damp woodlands of Manchuria.

Description: The aromatic root commonly grows to a length of 2 feet or more and is often divided at the end. The simple, glabrous stem bears, near the top, a whorl of three or five palmate compound leaves consisting of five oblong ovate, finely double serrated leaflets.

Uses: Ginseng is considered valuable for feverish and inflammatory illnesses; hemorrhage and for blood diseases. Women also take it for everything from normalizing menstruation to easing childbirth. Ginseng promotes both physical and mental vigor.

Resveratrol

Grapes used to refine Resverterol History: Recent research has shown that

It may have positive cardiac protective effects.

It has become a popular health supplement as a result.

Family Name: Wine Grapes

Botanical Name(s): White Hellebore extract Popular Name(s): Resvesterol

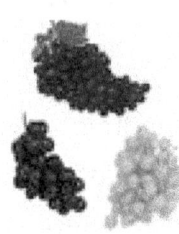

Parts Used: In grapes, Resvesterol is found primarily in the skin, and in muscadine grapes in the seeds. The amount found in grape skins also varies with the grape cultivar, its geographic origin, and exposure to fungal infection. The amount of fermentation time a wine spends in contact with grape skins is an important determinant of its Resvesterol content.

Habitat: Wine grape growing

regions everywhere Description:

Resvesterol was originally isolated by Takaoka from the roots of white hellebore in 1940, and later, in 1963, from the roots of Japanese knotweed. However, it attracted wider attention only in 1992, when its presence in wine was suggested as the explanation for the cardio protective effects of wine.

The mechanisms of Resvesterol's apparent effects on life extension are not fully understood; but they appear to mimic several of the biochemical effects of calorie restriction. A new report indicates that Resvesterol activates Sertuin 1 and PGC-1a, and improves functioning of the mitochondria. Other research calls into question the theory connecting Resvesterol, SIRT1, and calorie restriction.

Uses:

Thought to be useful for life extension, cancer prevention, and athletic performance

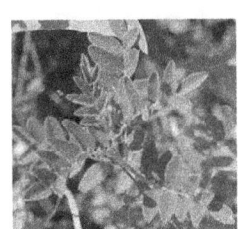

Astragalus Propinquus Family Name: Fabaceae

Botanical Name(s): Astragalus Membranaceus

Popular Name(s): Milk Vetch, Huang Qi, Milk Vetch root, Goat's Horn, Green Dragon, Yellow Emperor.

Parts Used: Roots

Habitat: Astragalus is indigenous to the northern and eastern parts of China and some areas of Mongolia.

Description: Astragalus Membranaceus is a sprawling perennial legume, about 16 inches high. Astragalus Membranaceus has a hairy stem, leaves made up of 12-18 leaflets and aromatic flowers.

Uses: Astragalus Membranaceus is widely used in traditional Chinese medicine and has proved its positive influence on human health. Astragalus is the primary herb used in Chinese medicines to tone the immune system of the lungs. It is useful for conditions of immune deficiency that leads to spontaneous sweating.

A drug extracted from a plant is used in Chinese medicine to help immune cells fight HIV which raises the possibility of slowing the ageing process in other parts of our bodies.

The method hinges upon telomeres - caps of repetitive DNA found at the ends of chromosomes. These get shorter as cells age and are thought to affect the cell's lifespan.

The caps can be rebuilt with an enzyme called telomerase, and some people have suggested it might be possible to extend human life by boosting telomerase production - though this has never been tested.

Now Rita Effros, at the University of California, in Los Angeles has used a drug that boosts telomerase to enhance the immune response to viruses.

The Importance of Regular exercise

Recent studies show more and more that one of the most powerful anti-aging things you can do for your body is regular exercise--even for the elderly.

My Dad is 90 years old this year, and he walks a mile each day, does sit ups, and uses arm weights. As you can guess--he is pretty active for his age.

A few years ago my Mom developed a severe case of Rheumatoid Arthritis.

Since she was very restricted in movement and couldn't exercise he lost body weight and started deteriorating fast.

If not for new drugs which can cure Rheumatoid Arthritis I think she would have died quickly. However, she did get treatment and started a new exercise regimen and is very healthy now for an 86 year old.

Information from an article on the benefits of exercise:

> The current broad guidelines from governmental and health organizations call for 150 minutes of moderate exercise per week to build and maintain health and fitness. But whether that amount of exercise represents the least amount that someone should do — the minimum recommended dose — or the ideal amount has not been certain.
>
> Scientists also have not known whether there is a safe upper limit on exercise, beyond which its effects become potentially dangerous; and whether some intensities of exercise are more effective than others at

prolonging lives. So the new studies, both of which were published last week in JAMA Internal Medicine, helpfully tackle those questions. In the broader of the two studies, researchers with the National Cancer Institute, Harvard University and other

institutions gathered and pooled data about people's exercise habits from six large, ongoing health surveys, winding up with information about more than 661,000 adults, most of them middle-aged.

Using this data, the researchers stratified the adults by their weekly exercise time, from those who did not exercise at all to those who worked out for 10 times the current recommendations or more (meaning that they exercised moderately for 25 hours per week or more).

Then they compared 14 years' worth of death records for the group. They found that, unsurprisingly, the people who did not exercise at all were at the highest risk of early death. But those who exercised a little, not meeting the recommendations but doing something, lowered their risk of premature death by 20 percent. Those who met the guidelines precisely, completing 150 minutes per week of moderate exercise, enjoyed greater longevity benefits and 31 percent less risk of dying during the 14-year period compared with those who never exercised.

The sweet spot for exercise benefits, however, came among those who tripled the recommended level of exercise, working out moderately, mostly by walking, for 450 minutes per week, or a little more than an hour per day. Those people were 39 percent less likely to die prematurely than people who never exercised. At that point, the benefits plateaued, the researchers found, but they never significantly declined.

Those few individuals engaging in 10 times or more the recommended exercise dose gained about the same reduction in mortality risk as people who simply met the guidelines. They did not gain significantly more health bang for all of those additional hours spent sweating. But they also did not increase their risk of dying young.

Section B: Long Lived Diets and Lifestyles

The Worlds Longest Lived Communities

I've avoided the subject of the best longevity diets for years since there are thousands of diets out there and I didn't feel I had anything new to present on the subject.

However, I recently spent more time reading about the lifestyles of very long lived persons and decided that the examples they and their communities represent needed to be shown to the world.

There have been many previous researchers and writers on the subject on healthily diets, but I thought my perspective on longevity might be unique since I focus mainly on successful lifestyles….and diet is part of the lifestyle.

The first thing I did in my research was to narrow down choices for the best longest lived communities to study.

My criteria for picking long lived communities were several:

- An unusually high proportion of the population is over one hundred years
- The community has a well defined culture
- Sufficient population so that lifestyles and eating habits are a common "Standard" model
- Fairly isolated communities which haven't been too "contaminated" by Western Cultures

The result was a decision to focus on these four communities around the world:

- Okinawa, Japan- This island has a very healthy lifestyle and has been extensively studied for their longevity. Estimate 1.3 million population 2015.

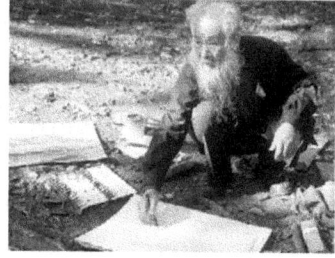

- The Republic of Abkhazia next to southern Russia. Population of 243,000 in 2012 census. A 1970 census had established Abkhazia, then an autonomous region within Soviet Georgia, as the longevity capital of the world. Very many persons over 100 years of age and even into 120- 130 age range.

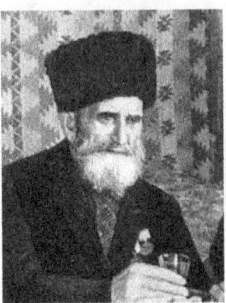

- Vilcabamba, Ecuador-This small community in the mountains of Ecuador is also known as "The Valley of Longevity". Population around 7,000 persons and a very high proportion of persons living to 130-140 years old

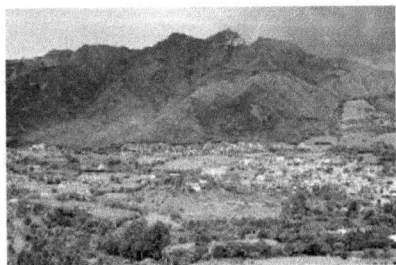

- The Hunza People of Pakistan-In far northern Pakistan at an elevation of 8,200 feet have many people over one hundred and persons who are 130-150 years old. An estimated population of 60,000

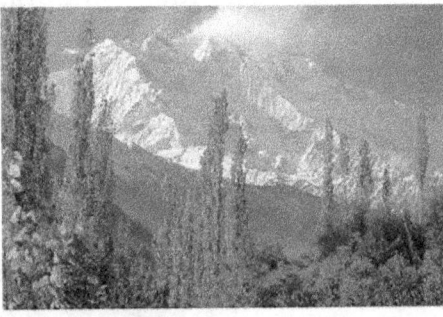

The materials in this Section B is taken from the Book:

"Diets and Lifestyles of the World's Oldest Persons"

In this book we are only reviewing the introductory information and summary tables.

The full book gives a lot more details on the lifestyles and diets along with recommendations to follow for healthly eating and even recipes for common foods these communities eat.

You can order a copy at: http://mkettingtonbooks.com

Comparisons of Lifestyle Factors:

Here is a matrix of both cultural and dietary factors. These factors are rated (High-Medium-Low) Types of foods are also provided in the Diet Table.

<u>Lifestyle Factors</u>

Description	Okinawa	Abkhazia	Vilcabamba	Hunzas
Exercise	*High*	*High*	*Medium*	*Very High*
Naturally Pure Water	*Medium*	*High*	*High*	*High*
Sense of Community	*High*	*High*	*High*	*High*
Happiness	*High*	*High*	*High*	*High*
Spiritual Practices & Inner Peace	*High*	*High*	*High*	*High*
Respect for Elderly	*High*	*High*	*High*	*High*

Dietary Factors/Foods

Description	Okinawa	Abkhazia	Vilcabamba	Hunzas
Vegetables	High-Sweet Potatos, Goya (bitter melon), Shima Rakkyo, Okra, Handama, Carrots, radish, marrow, onions, carrots, cabbage and leafy greens, Soya, squash	High- string beans, corn, cabbage, tomatoes, spinach, celery, dill, onions, spring onions, coriander, mint, basil, tarragon and parsley	High-Potatos, Mayoko, Payoko	High-Tomatoes, onions, garlic, spinach, turnips, carrots, pumpkins, cabbage, and cauliflower
Legumes	High	High	High	High-beans, lentils
Meat/Fat	Low-Pork	Low-Lamb	Low	Minimal
Grains	Rice	Buckwheat	High-Trigo (Wheat), Rice	wheat, barley, buckwheat, corn, millet, alfalfa, and rye
Fish	Low	Low	Low	Minimal
Fruits	High-Watermellon, Pineapple, Mango, Papaya, Passion Fruit, Shiikwa	High-Apples, cherry plums, barberries, blackberries, pomegranates, green grapes, tomatoes	High-oranges, blackberries, papayas, bananas, figs, avocados, Citroen, Granadias	High- mulberries, apricots, apples, cucumbers, grapes, peaches, cherries and some melons
Nuts	Pine nuts	Achapa, Walnuts	High-macadamia nuts, almonds	Almonds, Beachnuts, Walnuts, Flax
Special Bread		High-Limit Bread		High-Hunza Bread
Sugars	Sugarcane (Unrefined)	Honey, Sugarbeets	Panela-(Unrefined Sugarcane)	Honey
Other Common Foods		Yogurt, Garlic	Quinoa	Yogurt
Common Herbs		Saffron, Licorice		
Common Drinks	High-Tumeric Tea	High-Tea, Mountain Waters	High-Mountain Waters (Glacial Milk)	High-Mountain Waters
Number of DailyMeals				Two

From the above tables comparing lifestyles and diets here are my recommendations for the Longevity Diet which is taken from these real world examples:

1. Drink Pure Water--but not just bottled water but water with appropriate nutrients like the mountain streams provide to the long lived communities.
2. None of these communities are pure vegetarians but they all have very low levels of meat and fish--just because their traditional diets are oriented that way. Meat and Fish comprises only 1-3% of their daily diets
3. Two communities-- the Abkhazians and Hunzas eat natural grain, low fat, and high protein breads with fruit and nuts added. These are Limit Breads for the Abkhazians, and Hunza Breads for the Hunzas.
4. Several of the communities have lots of home grown fruits--of a variety of types. Eat lots of fruit.
5. Sugars are all natural or unrefined sugars whether from honey or from various types of fruits, or sugarcane.
6. They all consume high levels of legumes and vegetables. These types of food are the large majorities of their diets. (Greater than 65%)
7. The number of meals daily are only stated for the Hunzas who regularly eat two large meals daily. My research didn't tell me the number of meals in the other communities.

The Effect of Lifestyle Factors:

In the lifestyle factors table you can see a lot of parallels to the 10 Principles of Personal Longevity.

The principle longevity lifestyle factors I found from my research include:

- Lots of daily exercise--This ties into my previous research that exercise is one of the most critical factors in long term health.
- Naturally Pure Water with mountain nutrients-This was a surprise to me since I've heard others tout the benefits of water but never really gave it much serious consideration
- A strong Sense of Community- The community and happiness factors both illustrate the need for purpose and happiness to make our lives more fulfilling
- Overall Happiness

- Spiritual Practices & Inner Peace--A critical factor I've been teaching for years having earlier found that almost all super centenarians have these attributes which I believe help bring a spiritual blueprint of health down into our bodies
- Respect for Elderly--This relates a lot to the Principle of Life Purpose. People need meaning in their lives to go on living and being respected and asked for advice as an elderly person is important in making their lives worthwhile.

If you have read any of my other books on Longevity you will realize that these lifestyle factors are all part of what we already teach. They show some real world examples which further validate our 10 Principles approach.

Section C: Weight and Exercise

One final section we will cover under the physical body is that there are some misconceptions about ideal weights and exercise needed to promote longevity.

The following is a BMI chart (Body Mass Index)

According to this chart—and accepted guidelines—a BMI of over 25 is unhealthy and over 30 is obese and very unhealthy.

However, several studies on longevity suggest that the thresholds are different:

The best estimates of the association between body mass index (BMI) and mortality suggest that the mortality risk from excess body weight increases from a BMI of 25 but isn't substantial until BMI exceeds 32 or 35.

In fact it's the people that are overweight but below a BMI of 32 who are likelier to live longer. Those who are underweight are likely to have shorter lives.

This is an area of research we are still learning more about but we already see some contradictions to commonly held beliefs about weight and it's relationship to longevity.

Minimal Exercise Requirements

Now it is true that you need at least <u>ninety minutes of aerobic exercise every week</u> to promote body stability—especially as you get older.

I find that doing more like three to four hours of aerobic exercise each week helps keep me toned and with reasonable endurance.

Chapter Summary

You should read up on more books which talk about herbal supplements for health and choose to take ones which seem right for you.

You should also look carefully at the data about the Diet's and Lifestyles of the World's Oldest Persons and apply what they do to your life.

Also, make sure you have a regular exercise program to keep fit and maintain your body

After I covered all of the subjects which have an effect on long term health, then I realized there is one more topic which becomes extremely important when your body is ready to live a long time:

ACCIDENTS

10.0 Using Your Intuition for Safety

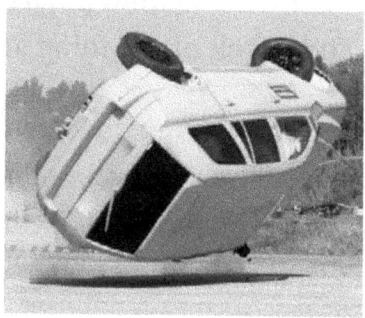

The ninth principle of personal longevity has to do with using your intuition to keep you safe.

Once you learn how to keep yourself healthy and your body young then accidents will become the biggest long term threat which may result in you becoming maimed or killed.

It is also interesting to note that the US Navy has written a field manual in 2017 to help Marines develop and use their intuition for safety in the field.

Long lived persons interviewed also have a belief that they have had at least one spiritual experience—maybe more than one which "saved them" from an accident which would have severely hurt them or killed them.

The ability to avoid accidents is a learned one.

Part of the spiritual development process can be to expand your "time sense" to detect danger before it happens. This can be from a few seconds before a car goes through an intersection to weeks, months, or years involving major life events.

In my own life I've experienced numerous times where I was saved by some "Spiritual Force" from a major accident or death.

Some of my accident avoidance experience clearly had a paranormal or spiritual component. The one that comes to mind the most is my "almost mugged" experience.

I would have definitely walked right into the muggers if my body hadn't sent me this urgent signal that

I had to urinate. I just couldn't go forward. When I tried twice I was stopped each time. Then the muggers came out from behind pillars and started walking towards us. This was when my friend and I took off running and got away.

Some persons experience pre-cognitive dreams where they dream of a terrible event happening to them or others. Later the event does happen. I remember a few years ago I had five or more dreams over months about different tropical beach resorts. Then the water all receded and later came in as a huge wave. This was all prior to the Indian Ocean Tsunami. The dreams stopped after the event.

Another example happened to me during August of 1998. My wife and I decided to send her and our kids to visit her mother in Barcelona, Spain.

I was waiting for a contract to close; so the plan was for me to buy a ticket separately, and meet them there during early September. When I started to call the travel agent to book my ticket I had a terrible feeling of fear about taking the flight.

I tried two other times to book the ticket during the week for a September 2nd departure, and each time I got the same strong feelings of fear and death.

I have always prayed, and tried to guard myself mentally to avoid disasters, so finally I took the warning seriously and decided not to go at all. This was very difficult to do since I really wanted to see my wife and kids, and this meant I would be home alone for a month.

Work wasn't an excuse either, since I wasn't doing any really heavy contract work at the time and could have easily taken the time off.

I called my wife and told her my decision, and she was surprised, but agreed for me to follow my instincts.

On September 2nd the Swissair disaster occurred on a plane leaving Kennedy airport in New York, which crashed in Newfoundland Canada with all lives lost.

I would not have originally been booked on that flight, but could have easily ended up on it since I was due to fly through Kennedy airport, and any delay might have caused me to switch planes.

I will never know for sure, but this was a very strong warning.

I should also mention that for several years before this event I had strong feelings that I would be killed in the near future. After the Swissair crash happened those feelings ended.

Since the future is only a probability, you can make decisions to allow you to avoid the accident and therefore change the future.

An exercise in learning how to avoid accidents:

- Go through a 5-10 minute relaxation exercise to calm you down and center your mind.
- Pick a trip you plan to take, or an event you plan to attend within the next year.
- Now imagine yourself on that trip or being at that event.
- Start feeling what is going on. For instance if it's a plane ride, how are the other passengers, the weather, the arrival, and trip to your final destination?
- Visualize all of these events happening while you are there.
- Now feel the emotions you would have at the time like fear or happiness.
- Go through the entire trip or event like this—being on the trip, doing all the activities and now returning.
- Finally, do the whole event or trip again in your mind's eye and see if you have the same feelings you did before during that time period.
- If you are like me, you may sense strong danger if something bad will happen.
- All I can advise you is if you do get a strong impression you should follow your intuition.

You can learn more about prophecy, it's history, and more exercises in my book "Prophecy: A History and How to Guide".

11.0 Implementing the Ten Principles In Your Life

There is a lot more to know than you can learn in this book about how to implement long term health and extended longevity in your life.

This book only provides a sampling of learning about longevity. You really need training or consulting to fully implement the ten longevity principles.

In my Personal Longevity consulting and training we offer a variety of services to help people with implementing the ten principles:

- One on one consulting to identify issues and blockages to implementing these practices
- The Personal Longevity Program online training which consists of over 60 hours of videos, audios, eBooks, exercises, and much more. Students completing this online training also receive a certificate as being a "Personal Longevity Program Certified Practitioner".
- Group training courses to teach these principles in person with in depth exercises and using many of the online materials.

Here are some of the steps we also use to help clients develop personal longevity implementation plans:

- During our initial one on one assessments, clients answers various questions for our profile spreadsheet. These answers help rank their status with different longevity criteria.
- We also provide a couple of worksheets to plan which specific practices make sense for the client to start as part of their implementation process.
- Also, we provide a scheduling worksheet so you can schedule what you will do when.
- Finally, we provide follow-up support including a blog and webinars to answer questions from clients and provide additional advice on how to proceed with living the ten principles of personal longevity in their lives.

12.0 Summary

One of the things that has really told me I'm on the right track with the ten principles of personal longevity is that so many other people have expressed similar concepts in their own ways.

I recently saw a presentation by a holistic healer who on her own had also identified the importance of synchronization between what she called the "spirit, mind, and body".

Another example is the seven beliefs below which come from an entirely different source but you will see the similarities to my holistic philosophical approach:

Seven Beliefs to Help Life Extension

Ben Abba has recently made some interesting claims on his website about longevity:

He says that by remote viewing and other techniques he was able to find numerous persons around the world aged 150 years or more.

He also says that he found two persons of 2800 years of age and was able to interview one of them in the Eastern Mediterranean at length.

Here is a list of seven items that Ben Abba generated from his interviews with the "immortals" he met. He believes this list will keep anyone onto the road to immortality.

Belief in a Creator

There are several beliefs that are required to extend our lives. However I have noticed a particular belief that is critical to accomplishing both. The most important belief to extending our lives is a belief in a supreme being aka God. If you are stuck in believing that humans are mere biological machines that appeared on earth by accident, immortality is not for you. If you can wake up to the fact that humans are also spiritual beings, then you can lift yourself out of becoming planetary road kill and advance onto the path of becoming immortal. All of the "immortals" that I met had a personal relationship with God.

Belief in Life Extension

The second most important belief necessary to extend our lives is the conviction that extending our lives is not only possible, but it is our right as spiritual beings. The mind does control matter; and there are millions of examples to prove this. If you have the necessary beliefs your spirit will automatically frame your lifestyle into extending your life; even to the point of becoming an immortal. All of the "immortals" that I met only believed in life and refused to believe in death.

Love

Love is the most powerful energy in our universe and is also the "food" our souls need to grow, to evolve, and to accomplish powerful things. Love comes in many forms and is expressed in many ways. From what I have learned so far giving love or receiving love feeds our soul. All of the "immortals" that I have met have loving family members, caring friends, and love life in general.

Attitude

Once you can get yourself to comprehend the "beliefs" that will extend your life your attitude about living life becomes important. If you are still struggling with your beliefs, then try to master that. You do not need to live life in total denial, but wearing the rose colored glasses as often as you can, to see the positive in life does help tremendously. All of the "immortals" that I met had a very positive outlook on life and fully believed their minds did much more than control their bodies.

Energy

More important than food and exercise for human survival is energy. Our bodies require many different kinds of energy to perform all of the incredible tasks that humans perform, including survival. And while it is true that love, food, air and exercise give our physical bodies' energy, they give our spiritual bodies energy too.

All of the "immortals" that I met made it a point to get out into the sun at least once a day, talk to someone at least once a day, and most importantly share a meal with someone at least once a day.

Exercise

Our physical bodies do require some kind of exercise every day. All of the "immortals" that I have met walked every day; sometimes for many miles.

Diet

As we all suspect, what we put into our bodies determines our survival. Despite popular belief, all of the "immortals" that I have met are not 100% vegetarians.

Instead they all eat a balance diet of vegetables, grains, a little fruit and some meat. However the animal protein they do eat is primarily mutton, fish, and pheasant; making up 10% to 20% of their diets.

All of the "immortals" that I have researched drank one or two glasses of wine, between meals, every day

****

Notice the similarities in the above guidelines to the ten principles which I developed through my experience and research.

Other holistic professionals I talk with also immediately "get it". This is either because they have thought the same things for many years, or because they quickly recognize the truth of what I'm saying.

I really believe in the importance of these ten principles and wish all of you God's love and blessings to live a long, healthy, and happy life.

If you want to learn more about the longevity lifestyle we teach please go to my website: http://personal-longevity.com

All the Best,

Marty Ettington

February 2017

13.0 Bibliography

1. Yogananda, Paramahansa. *Autobiography of a Yogi.* s.l.: Self Realization Fellowship, 1946.
2. Wong, Eva. *The Taoist Immortals.* s.l.: Shambala Publications, Inc., 2001.
3. Various. *The Holy Bible.* s.l.: KJV, NIS, IS, RSV.
4. Taimni, I. K. *The Science of Yoga.* Madras India/London England: The Theosophical Publishing House, 1975.
5. Smith, Malcolm. *How I Learned to Meditate.* s.l.: Logos International, 1977.
6. Schenkman, Richard. *The 14,000 Year Old Man.* 2007.
7. Powell, A. E. *The Mental Body.* 1970: The Thesophical Press.
8. Peace, Foundation for Inner. A Course in Miracles. *A Course in Miracles.* [Online] Foundation for Inner Peace. [Cited: 11 9, 2008.] http://www.acim.org/index.html.
9. Orr, Leonard. *Breaking the Death Habit.* Berkely, Ca.: Frog Limited, 1970.
10. Olson, Stuart Alve. *Qigong Teachings of a Taoist Immortal.* s.l.: Harper Arts Press, 2002.
11. Mulcahy, Russell. *The Highlander.* 1986.
12. Mickaharic, Draja. *Immortality.* s.l.: Lulu, Inc., 2007.
13. —. *Immortality.*
14. Liebers, Arthur. *Relax with Yoga.* [Online] [Cited: 11 11, 2008.] http://www.sacred-texts.com/hin/rwy/rwy09.htm.
15. Leadbeater, C. W. *The Chakras.* s.l.: The Theosophical Publishing House, 1973.
16. King, Godfre Ray. *The Magic Presence.* s.l.: Saint Germain Press, Inc., 1963.
17. Kelder, Peter. *Ancient Secret of the Fountain of Youth: Book 1.* s.l.: Doubleday, 1/20/1998.
18. Heinlein, Robert. *Methuselah's Children.* 1941.
19. George M. Gould, M.D., Walter L. Pyle, M.D. Longevity: Effect of Class-Influences, Occupation. *Anomalies and Curiosities of Medicine.* [Online] http://www.enotalone.com/article/14903.html.

20. Gaze, Hary. *How to Live Forever with Golden Rules for Successful Living.* s.l.: Kessinger Publishing, 1905.
21. Gaze, Harry. *How To Live Forever With Golden Rules For Successful Living.* 1904.
22. Edwards, Frank. *Stranger than Science.* 1960.
23. Bharat B. Aggarwal (Editor), Shishir Shishodia. *Resveratrol in Health and Disease.* s.l.: CRC Press, 2006.
24. Authors, Many. *The Holy Bible--NIV, KJV, NIS, LB Versions.* Various.
25. Asanaro. *Seamm Jasani 50 MOvements for Eternal Youth from Ancient Tibet.* s.l.: Tarcher/Putnam, 2003.
26. Anderson, Poul. *The Boat of a Million Years.* s.l.: Tom Doherty Associates, Inc., 1989.
27. Abba, Ben. *How to Live to 150 or More.* [Online] 2008. http://howtoliveto150.com/.
28. *The Chakras.* [Online] [Cited: 10 30, 2008.] http://www.kheper.net/topics/chakras/chakras.htm.
29. Telomeres. *Wikipedia.* [Online] http://en.wikipedia.org/wiki/Telomere.
30. Tai Chi Chuan. *Wikipedia.* [Online] [Cited: 11 3, 2008.] http://en.wikipedia.org/wiki/Tai_chi_chuan.
31. Rheumatoid Arthritis Health Center. *www.webmd.com.* [Online] http://www.webmd.com/rheumatoid-arthritis/features/rheumatoid-arthritis-keeping-positive-outlook.
32. *On the Physics and Phenomenology of Time.* [Online] [Cited: 11 5, 2008.] http://www.goertzel.org/papers/timepap.html.
33. Life Expectancy. *Wikipedia.* [Online] [Cited: 11 2, 2008.] http://en.wikipedia.org/wiki/Life_expectancy.
34. Li Ching-Yun Dead; Gave his age as 197. *The New York Times.* May 6, 1933.
35. Kundalini. *The Mystica.* [Online] [Cited: 11 3, 2008.] http://www.themystica.com/mystica/articles/k/kundalini.html.
36. Holosync. *Centerpointe Research Institute.* [Online] [Cited: 11 3, 2008.] http://www.centerpointe.com/.
37. *Ginseng.* [Online] http://www.herbsguide.net/ginseng.html.
38. Fo-ti-tieng. *Fo-ti-tieng.* [Online] [Cited: 10 28, 2008.] http://www.herbsguide.net/fo-ti-tieng.html.
39. Astragalus_propinquus. *Wikipedia.* [Online] [Cited: 11 17, 2008.] http://en.wikipedia.org/wiki/Astragalus_propinquus.

40. A Gallery of Chinese Immortals. *A Gallery of Chinese Immortals.* [Online] [Cited: 11 10, 2008.] http://www.angelfire.com/in4/alchemy2084/giles.html.
41. REYNOLDS, GRETCHEN. *The Right Dose of Exercise for a Long Life.* 2015.

14.0 Index

A Course in Miracles, 75 *A Positive Outlook*, 61 Abd el Aziz el Habachi, 33 Acupuncture, 73, 109
Acupuncture meridians, 109
Animals, 130
Anterior Nervous System, 72 Antisa Khvichava, 30
ARTHUR LIEBERS, 125
Ascended Immortals, 37
Astragalus propinquus, 143
Attitude, 163
Baba Harainsingh, 25
Babaji, 38, 56
Bandhas, 125
Belief in a Creator, 162 Belief in Life Extension, 162 Ben Abba, 161
Bhartriji, 38 Biblical Persons
Adam, 35
Enoch, 36
Enosh, 35
Jared, 36
Kenan, 35
Lamech, 36
Mahalalel, 36
Methuselah, 36
Moses, 36
Noah, 36
Seth, 35
Biblical Quotes Relating to Stillness, 67
Big Bang, 65
Biological Immortality, 134

Black Holes, 66
Calorie Restriction, 136
Cell lines, 135
Cellular Regeneration, 123
Chakra, 109 Chakras
3rd eye, 110
Crown Chakra, 110
Heart, 110
Root, 110
Sacrum/Feeling, 110
Solar Plexus, 110
Throat, 110
Charlie Smith, 20
Chen Jun, 33
Christianity, 67
Count St. Germain, 122 crown chakra, 111
Daily affirmations for Eternal Youth, 59
David Kinnison, 19
Death Urge, 56
Devraha Baba, 26
Diet, 163
Drakenberg, 22
Elizabeth Yorath, 25 Enabling Your Life Urge, 55 Energy, 163
Energy Body, 73
Exercise, 163
Exercises in Unconditional Love, 97 Eye of Revelation, 114
Five Tibetan Rites, 114 Fo-ti-tieng, 141
Fountain of Youth, 115

G. Stanley, 22 *Gentle Boabom*, 116
    Ginseng, 141
Golden Rules to Live Forever, 57 Great
    White Brotherhood, 37 Great White
    Lodge, 37
Harry Gaze, 57
Hatha Yoga, 125
Henry Jenkins, 24
Holy Spirit, 68
How to Live Forever, 57 Hydra, 135
Implementing the ten principles, 159
    Importance of Stillness, 69 Individual
    plant specimens, 130 Ivan Yorath, 25
Javier Pereira, 24
Jeanne Louise Calment, 20 John Rovin, 25
Jonas Warren, 23
Joseph Surrington, 23
Katherine Fitzgerald, 21
Kentigren, 25
Kundalini, 111, 127
Leonard Orr, 55
Leonard Orr:, 55
Li Ching-yun, 28
LI CHING-YUN, 27, 28
Life Without a Purpose, 45 *Living
    in Awareness*, 53 Long Lived
    Communities
Okinawa, Japan, 146
The Hunza People of Pakistan, 147
    The Republic of Abkhazia, 146
    Vilcabamba, Ecuador, 147
Long Lived Persons
Abd-el-Aziz-Habachi, 33
Anthony Senish, 19
Antisa Khvichava, 30

Baba Harainsingh, 25
Butler, 20
Charlie Smith, 20
Chen Jun, 33
Colonel Thomas Winslow, 21
David Kinnison, 19
Dr. William Hotchkiss, 21
Drakenberg, 22
Eglebert Hoff, 20
Elizabeth Yorath, 25
G. Stanley, 22 Henry Jenkins, 24 Ivan
    Yorath, 25 Javier Pereira, 24 Jean
    Effingham, 21 Jeanne Calment, 20
    John Rovin, 25 Jonas Warren, 23
Joseph Surrington, 23
Katherine Fitzgerald, 21
Kentigren, 25
LI CHING-YUN, 27
Moloko Temo, 20
Mr. Evans, 21
Mrs. Eckelston, 21
Nestor, 33
Nicolas Petours, 20
Petratsh Zartan, 25
R. Glen, 19
Robert Lynch, 23
Sampson Skakoragaro, 22
Shirali Mislimov, 24
Thomas Parr, 22
Tiresias, 33
Trailanga Swami, 33
Turinah, 31
William Edwards, 23
Wizzardo (Siddha) Sayadaw U. Kowida, 32
Zaro Ağa, 23

14.0 Index

Love, 162
Love and Affection, 78 *Love and Friendship,* 81 *Love and Romance,* 83 *Love Defined Through Quotes,* 85 *Loving in the Now,* 100 meditation, 70, 116
Methuselah-World's oldest tree, 130
Moloko Temo, 20
My Heart Opening Experience, 104
Nestor, 33
Optimism, 61
Paths to Unconditional Love, 94 peace, 67, 68
Peter Kelder, 114
Petratsh Zartan, 25
Positive Outlook, 61
Qi, 118
Qigong, 118
Quantum Physics, 66
quietness, 68
Ram Dass, 92
Red Wine Extract, 136 Relax with Yoga, 125 <u>Resvesterol</u>, 142
Resvesterol, 136
Robert Lynch, 23
Sacred Fire, 121
Sampson Skakoragaro, 22
Seamm Jasani, 116
Setting Goals, 52
Shirali Mislimov, 24
Spiritual Connection, 65
Stillness, 66, 69
Tai Chi, 118
Tai chi chuan, 120 *Tai Chi Chuan,* 120
Taoist Immortals, 39
Chang Kuo, 40
Chung-li Ch'uan, 40
Han Hsiang Tzu, 41
Ho Hsien Ku, 42
Lan Ts'ai-ho, 42
Li T'ieh-kuai, 41
Lu Yen, 40
Peng-Tzu, 40
Ts'ao Kuo-chiu, 41
technological solution, 137
telomeres, 135, 136
The Mudras, 125
The Reality of Stillness, 65 The Seed of the Woman, 29
The Worlds Longest Lived Communities, 146 Theosophists, 73
Thomas Carn, 26
Thomas Parr, 22
Tiresias, 33
Trailanga Swami, 33
Turinah, 31
Unconditional Love:, 89 Victor H. Mair, 39 Violet Flame, 121, 122
Visualizing your Immortal Future, 62 Vital Forces, 109
What is Purpose?, 51
What is the goal of this love?, 95
Who you Really are, 49 William Edwards, 23
Xian, 39
Your Mission in Life, 49 Zaro Ağa, 23

www.ingramcontent.com/pod-product-compliance
Lightning Source LLC
Chambersburg PA
CBHW080519030426
42337CB00023B/4566